Comprehensive Lactation Consultant Exam Review

Comprehensive Lactation Consultant Exam Review

LINDA J. SMITH
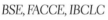
BSE, FACCE, IBCLC

JONES AND BARTLETT PUBLISHERS

Sudbury, Massachusetts

BOSTON   TORONTO   LONDON   SINGAPORE

World Headquarters
Jones and Bartlett Publishers
40 Tall Pine Drive
Sudbury, MA 01776
978-443-5000
info@jbpub.com
www.jbpub.com

Jones and Bartlett Publishers Canada
2406 Nikanna Road
Mississauga, Ontario
Canada L5C 2W6

Jones and Bartlett Publishers International
Barb House, Barb Mews
London W6 7PA
UK

ISBN: 0-7637-0920-4

Copyright © 2001 by Jones and Bartlett Publishers, Inc.

Library of Congress Cataloging-in-Publication Data

Smith, Linda J., 1946-
    Comprehensive lactation consultant exam review / Linda J. Smith.
        p. ; cm
    Includes bibliographical references.
    ISBN 0-7637-0920-4
    1. Breast Feeding—Examinations, questions, etc. 2. Lactation—Examinations, questions,
    etc. I. Title.
    [DNLM: 1. Breast Feeding—Examination Questions 2. Lacation—Examination
    Questions. 3. Lacation Disorders—Examination Questions. WS 18.2 S654c 2000]
    RJ216 .S56 2000
    613.2'69'076—dc21

                                                                00-037084

Production Credits
Chief Executive Officer: Clayton Jones
Chief Operating Officer: Don W. Jones, Jr.
Executive Vice President and Publisher: Tom Manning
V.P., Sales and Marketing: Paul Shepardson
V.P., College Editorial Director: Brian L. McKean
V.P., Managing Editor: Judith H. Hauck
V.P., Design and Production: Anne Spencer
Marketing Manager: Lynn Protasowicki
Acquisitions Editor: John Danielowich
Production Editor: Rebecca S. Marks
Editorial/Production Assistant: Christine Tridente
Director of Manufacturing and Inventory Control: Therese Bräuer
Cover Design: AnnMarie Lemoine
Design and Composition: The Clarinda Company
Printing and Binding: Courier
Cover printing: Courier

Enclosed CD-ROM photo credits:
Gregory Notestine, DDS: A124, A126, A129, A149, A150, A151, A152, A153, A155, A158
A167, A169, B124, B145, B149, B150, B151, B152, B154, B170, C124, C126, C127, C149,
C151, C152, C1269, C170, C171
Kathleen Hoover, M Ed, IBCLC: B153
Sarah Coulter Danner, CNM, CPNP, IBCLC: B125

Printed in the United States of America
04 03 02   10 9 8 7 6 5 4 3 2

Table of Contents

To Denny
Thank you for nurturing my dreams with your support,
shelter, and encouragement. Your wisdom, analytic skills,
and calm strength are my foundation and source of courage.

To Edwin, Hannah, and Carl
Thank you for the privilege of mothering you.
You changed my life forever and continue to fill
my inner place with joy, pride, and love.

Linda J. Smith, BSE, FACCE, IBCLC is an internationally known author, teacher, and lecturer and proud grandmother. Linda has worked in public health, hospital-based perinatal education, private practice, policy and political forums, professional teaching, and volunteer organizations to support, protect, and promote breastfeeding for nearly 30 years in 9 cities in 2 countries.

Linda is a founding/charter member of the International Board of Lactation Consultant Examiners and was project leader for the initial Role Delineation Study, Practice Analysis. She served on the 1985 Exam Committee, developed the first Proctor's Manual, and was Chief Proctor for the first certifying exam administration.

Linda was also a founding/charter Board member of the International Lactation Consultant Association, serving on its Board of Directors from 1985 to 1988 and 1995 to 1997. She later led and continues to be involved in development of global standards for professional lactation education.

Linda is Director and co-owner of *Bright Future Lactation Resource Centre* in Dayton, Ohio, which develops and publishes a wide range of educational and promotional materials for breastfeeding care providers. BFLRC is on the Internet at *www.BFLRC.com.*

ACKNOWLEDGEMENTS

This book would not have been possible without my husband Denny's emotional support, financial shelter, and technical brilliance in computers. The roots of this book go back to the roots of the lactation consultant profession in the early 1980's, when Judy Good and Betty Ann Countryman of La Leche League International first floated the concept of the professional lactation consultant. Thank you, La Leche League International, for having the faith and courage to foster the development of a mid-level counselor who works collaboratively with mother support groups and health care professionals to support the breastfeeding mother-baby dyad.

Thanks to Editor John Danielowich at Jones and Bartlett who kept faith with this project (and with me) as the book changed and evolved into its present form. Special thanks goes to Rebecca Marks for her patience and creativity while guiding the book through production.

Thank you, Mary Riley Renard, RN, BSN, IBCLC—your wise oversight and editing of hundreds of exam questions helped me keep perspective and focus on the fundamental skills, knowledge, and attitudes essential for competent lactation consultant work. Your many years of experience with past IBLCE examinations brings special authenticity to these practice exams.

Special thanks are extended to the students who took the *Lactation Consultant Exam Preparation Course* taught through Lact-Ed, Inc. over the past 7 years. Although Lact-Ed, Inc. is no longer teaching courses, its spirit will be reborn through you, as the students of yesterday become the teachers of tomorrow. You all have taught me much about the process of learning about lactation.

I want to especially thank Peggy Loyd and Nancy Schweers. Peggy patiently listened to my insecurities as a new mother, building my confidence one phone call at a time. In addition to nurturing and inspiring me through crucial passages of my life, Nancy quietly, gently, and effectively advocated for breastfeeding and the unique role of the lactation consultant in political and public policy arenas in the United States and worldwide. She is a true unsung hero of the lactation consultant movement.

I am enormously grateful to the mothers and babies whose stories and photos bring life and realism to this book. I hope I've conveyed their collective persistence, courage, and strength. To Edwin, Hannah, and Carl—my now-adult children—thank you for teaching me how to mother and what breastfeeding is "really" all about. I am especially grateful to Hannah Boswell for allowing me to witness her skilled mothering of her daughter (my granddaughter) Carrie.

And lastly, I want to thank my husband Dennis for his financial support, faith in my abilities, and for prodding me into the Information

Age. The fundamental concepts and documents of the lactation consultant profession were born in the early 1980's on our Commodore 64 computer, which was cutting-edge technology at the time. Denny's technical expertise and support has been as fundamental to the creation of this profession and this book as mother's milk is to the growth of a healthy child. I simply can't fathom doing a project of this magnitude without modern computers and the Internet, and a live-in wizard whose patient nurturing support gives shape and form to my thoughts.

Comprehensive Lactation Consultant Exam Review is a well-referenced book and CD-ROM learning package that will help you review material that is tested on the international lactation consultant certification examination administered by the International Board of Lactation Consultant Examiners (IBLCE). From her perspective as a founding member of IBLCE and ILCA, Linda J. Smith provides 600 multiple-choice questions including 240 photographs arranged into three complete practice tests that conform to the 2000 exam blueprint published by IBLCE.

The chapters correspond to the disciplines listed for the IBLCE exam blueprint for the year 2000 and beyond. However, some common sub-topics that are not specifically itemized by IBLCE could fall into more than one category. Each sub-topic is included in only *one* category to avoid duplicating reading and references for that topic.

The recommended readings are the minimum needed for good understanding of the topic. Additional readings offer a broader or more in-depth look at the topics in the chapter. Examine the edition number of the references carefully, and use the most recent editions whenever possible. If one reference contradicts another, look carefully for the common ground, or examine the cited primary research on the topic. The exam will test the universal principles, not esoteric trivia.

Each chapter has an extensive bibliography and citations for the evidence-based and theory-driven material presented in each topic. In some cases, the entire research article can be downloaded from the journal's site on the Internet. In other cases, only the abstract is available online. Most medical libraries will provide access to a wide selection of the journals cited.

❒ *Knowledge* areas are easily found in the recommended readings and bibliographies.
❒ *Skills* are learned through experience, preferably supervised, and indirectly tested in the sample questions, especially the questions with accompanying photographs.
❒ *Attitudes* are difficult to test with a paper-and-pencil examination, yet central to effective breastfeeding care. Listening to mothers' concerns and experiences is vital to understanding the supportive attitudes that emerge in the sample questions.

The sample questions may include signs and symptoms of various diseases, therapeutic treatments including antibiotics and other prescription medications, and other information related to the overall health or medical condition of the lactating mother or breastfed child.

Inclusion of this information DOES NOT imply that the lactation consultant, on the basis of IBCLC certification alone, is qualified or

legally allowed to diagnose *medical conditions* or recommend, prescribe or determine *medical treatments* of the mother or child. Although this book will help prepare for the IBLCE exam, no guarantees of passing the IBLCE exam are expressed or implied.

This book is intended to augment in-person lactation management or exam preparation courses, not replace them. Students in lactation management courses often find that coursework focuses their study, validates existing knowledge, and identifies weak areas. The book can also be used as a guide for self-study or formation of study groups.

The CD-ROM contains the full-color pictures needed to answer the questions in the clinical section of the practice tests. The images depict situations commonly encountered in lactation consultant practice, and are used to test the candidate's clinical judgment.

To learn more about IBLCE certification, contact the International Board of Lactation Consultant Examiners, 7309 Arlington Blvd., Suite 300, Falls Church, VA 22042-3215, phone (703) 560-7330; fax (703) 560-7332; e-mail *iblce@erols.com*; internet *www.IBLCE.org*. IBLCE maintains regional offices in Australia and Germany.

Comprehensive Lactation Consultant
Exam Review

1

Maternal and Infant Anatomy

In the exam blueprint[1], 19 to 33 questions are dedicated to maternal and infant anatomy, specifically breast and nipple anatomy and infant oral anatomy.

SUBTOPICS INCLUDED IN THIS CATEGORY

1. Breast and nipple anatomy
   a. General development
   b. Changes during pregnancy
   c. Nipple variations
   d. Breast size variations
   e. Vascular, lymph, and nervous systems
2. Infant
   a. General, including embryology and fetal anatomy
   b. Gastrointestinal tract
   c. Head, neck, and oral anatomy
   d. Structures involved in suck-swallow-breathe

CORE READING

Black R, Jarman L, Simpson J. *Lactation Specialist Self-Study Modules #1-4.* Sudbury, MA: Jones & Bartlett Publishers; 1998: module #3, chap 1 A & C.

Lauwers J, Shinskie D. *Counseling the Nursing Mother.* 3rd ed. Sudbury, MA: Jones & Bartlett Publishers, 2000: chaps 6, 11, 13.

Lawrence RA, Lawrence RM. *Breastfeeding, a Guide for the Medical Profession.* 5th ed. St. Louis: Mosby; 1999: chaps 2, 3.

---

[1]All grid citations throughout this text are from the year 2000 Candidate's Guide.

Morbacher N. and Stock J. *The Breastfeeding Answer Book,* rev. ed. Schaumburg, IL: La Leche League International; 1997: chap 4.

Riordan J, Auerbach KG. *Breastfeeding and Human Lactation.* 2nd ed. Sudbury, MA: Jones & Bartlett Publishers; 1999: chap 4.

Wolf L, Glass R. *Feeding and Swallowing Disorders in Infancy.* Tucson, AZ: Therapy Skill Builders; 1992: chaps 1, 8.

Woolridge M. Anatomy of infant sucking. *Midwifery.* 1986; 2:164-171.

ADDITIONAL RESOURCES

Alexander JM, Grant AM, Campbell MJ. Randomized controlled trial of breast shells and Hoffman's exercises for inverted and non-protractile nipples. *Br Med J.* 1992;304:1030-1032.

Ardran GM, et al. A cineradiographic study of breastfeeding. *Br J Radiol.* 1958;31(363):156-162.

Bowen-Jones A, Thompson C, Drewett RF. Milk flow and sucking rates during breastfeeding. *Dev Med Child Neurol.* 1982;24:626-633.

Bu'Lock F, Woolridge MW, Baum JD. Development of coordination of sucking, swallowing, and breathing: ultrasound study of term and preterm infants. *Dev Med Child Neurol.* 1990;32:669-676.

Davis D, et al. Infant feeding practices and occlusal outcomes: a longitudinal study. *J Can Dent Assoc.* 1991;57(7):593-594.

Inoue N, Sakashita R, Kamegai T. Reduction of masseter muscle activity in bottle-fed babies. *Early Hum Dev.* 1995;42:185-193.

Ironside JW, Guthrie W. The galactocele: a light- and electron microscopic study. *Histopathology.* 1985;9:457-467.

Klaus MH. The frequency of suckling-neglected but essential ingredient of breast-feeding. *Obstet Gynecol Clin North Am.* 1987;14:623-633.

Labbok MH, Hendershot GE. Does breastfeeding protect against malocclusion? An analysis of the 1981 child health supplement to the National Health Interview Survey. *Am J Prev Med.* 1987;3(4):227-232.

Lipsitt LP, Reily BM, Butcher MJ, Greenwood MM. The stability and interrelationships of newborn sucking and heart rate. *Dev Psychobiol.* 1974;9(4):305-310.

Lombardino LJ, Stapell JB, Gerhardt KJ. Evaluating communicative behaviors in infancy. *J Pediatr Healthcare* 1987;1(5):240-246.

Love SM. *Dr. Susan Love's Breast Book.* 2nd ed. Reading, MA: Addison-Wesley; 1995:chap 1.

Lucas A, Lucas PJ, Baum JD. Pattern of milk flow in breastfed infants. *Lancet.* July 14, 1979; 8133-8134.

Mathew OP, Bhatia J. Sucking and breathing patterns during breast- and bottle-feeding in term neonates. *AJDC.* 1989;143:588-592.

Mathew OP. Science of bottle feeding. *Pediatrics.* 1991;119(4):511-519.

Morris S. In: Palmer MM, ed. *The normal acquisition of oral feeding skills: implications for assessment and treatment.* New York: Theraputic Media; 1982. Chaps 2-5.

Neifert M, De Marzo S, Seacat S, Young P, Leff M, Orleans M. The influence of breast surgery, breast appearance, and pregnancy-induced breast changes on lactation sufficiency as measured by infant weight gain. *Birth.* 1990;17(1):31-38.

Neifert, M. Breastfeeding after breast surgical procedure or breast cancer. *NAACOG's Clin Issues Perina Women's Health Nurs.* 1992;3(4):673-682.

Neifert, M, McDonough SL, Neville MC. Failure of lactogenesis associated with placental retention. *Am J Obste Gynecol.* 1981;140:477-478.

Neifert, M, Seacat JM, Jobe WE. Lactation failure due to insufficient glandular development. *Pediatrics.* 1985;76:832-828.

Netter FH. *Atlas of Human Anatomy.* Summit, NJ: Ciba-Geigy Corporation; 1989.

Neville MC, Neifert MR. *Lactation: Physiology, Nutrition and Breastfeeding.* New York: Plenum Press; 1983:chap 1-5.

Newton MR, Newton N. Relation of the let-down reflex to the ability to breastfeed. *Pediatrics.* 1950;5:726.

Restak R. *The Brain.* New York: Doubleday; 1979.

Righard L, Alade MO. Sucking technique and its effect on success of breastfeeding. *Birth.* December 1992;19(4):185-189.

Ross MW. *Back to the breast: retraining infant suckling patterns.* Chicago: La Leche League International; 1987: Lactaction Consultant Series, Unit 15.

Royal College of Midwives. *Successful Breastfeeding.* 2nd ed. London: Churchill Livingstone; 1991.

Shrago L, Bocar D. The infant's contribution to breastfeeding. *JOGNN,* 1990;19(3):209-215.

Smith W, et al. Physiology of sucking in the normal term infant using real-time ultrasound. *Radiology.* 1985;156:379.

Snyder JB. *Variation in Infant Palatal Structure* [master's thesis]. Sun Valley, CA: self published: 1995.

Spitz AM, Lee NC, Peterson HB. Treatment for lactation supression: little progress in one hundred years. *Am J Obstet Gynecol.* 1998 Dec;179(6): 1485-1490.

Weber F, et al. An ultrasonographic study of the organization of sucking and swallowing by newborn infants. *Dev Med Child Neurol.* 1986;28:19-24.

Widstrom AM, Thingstrom-Paulsson J. The position of the tongue during rooting reflexes elicited in newborn infants before the first suckle. *Acta Paediatr Scand.* 1993;82:281-283.

Widstrom AM, Wahlberg V, et al. Short-term effects of early suckling and touch of the nipple on maternal behavior. *Early Hum Dev.* 1990; 21:153-163.

Wilson JM, ed. *Oral-motor Function and Dysfunction in Children.* Chapel Hill, NC: University of North Carolina at Chapel Hill; 1977.

Woolridge M, et al. Individual patterns of milk intake during breastfeeding. *Early Hum Dev.* 1982;4:265-272.

Woolridge M. Anatomy of infant sucking. *Midwifery.* 1986;2:164-171.

Woolridge M, Baum, JD. The regulation of human milk flow. In: Lindblad BS. *Perinatal Nutrition.* Vol. 6. London: Academic Press; 1988.

2

Maternal and Infant Physiology and Endocrinology

In the exam blueprint, 19 to 33 questions are dedicated to maternal and infant physiology and endocrinology, specifically, hormones, milk production, infant bodily functions, including digestion etc. and fertility.

SUBTOPICS INCLUDED IN THIS CATEGORY

1. Maternal/female hormones—general
2. Milk production (milk synthesis—process)
    a. Lactogenesis and involution
    b. Relactation
    c. Induced lactation
3. Fertility
    a. Family planning, including Lactation Amenorrhea Method (LAM)
    b. Sexuality
    c. Breastfeeding during pregnancy; tandem nursing
4. Infant bodily functions, including digestion
    a. Placental nutrition to breastfeeding—evolution of infant nutrition
    b. Stool patterns; gut closure, gut microflora
    c. Process of suck-swallow-breathe

CORE READING

Black RF, Jarman L, Simpson J. *Lactation Specialist Self-Study Modules #1-4.* Sudbury, MA: Jones & Bartlett Publishers; 1998: module 2 chap 2 C & D, module 3 chap 1B, module 4 chap 2 A & B, chap 3 B & C.

Cregan MD, Hartmann PE. Computerized breast measurement from conception to weaning: clinical implications. *J Hum Lact.* 1999;15(2):89-96.

Daly SEJ, Hartmann PE: Infant demand and milk supply. Part 1: Infant demand and milk supply in lactating women. *J Hum Lact.* 1995;11:21-26.

Daly SEJ, Hartmann, PE: Infant demand and milk supply. Part 2: The short-term control of milk synthesis in lactating women. *J Hum Lact.* 1995;11:27-31.

Lauwers J, Shinskie D. *Counseling the Nursing Mother.* 3rd ed. Sudbury, MA: Jones & Bartlett Publishers; 2000: chaps 6, 10, 14, 20.

Lawrence RA. *Breastfeeding, a Guide for the Medical Profession.* 5th ed. St. Louis: Mosby; 1999: chaps 3, 6, 18, 19.

Morbacher N, Stock J. *The Breastfeeding Answer Book.* rev ed. Schaumburg, IL: La Leche League International, 1997: chaps 2, 3, 7, 8, 16, 17, 18.

Riordan J, Auerbach KG. *Breastfeeding and Human Lactation.* 2nd ed. Sudbury, MA: Jones & Bartlett Publishers; 1999: chaps 10, 21.

Stuart-Macadam P, Dettwyler KA. *Breastfeeding: Biocultural Perspectives.* New York: Aldine De Gruyter; 1995: chaps 8, 11.

Sutherland A, Auerbach KG. *Relactation and Induced Lactation.* Wayne, NJ: Avery Publishing Group; 1985: Lactation Consultant Series Unit 1.

ADDITIONAL RESOURCES

_____. *The Womanly Art of Breastfeeding.* 6th rev ed. Schaumburg, IL: La Leche League International; 1997.

Akre J, ed. *Infant Feeding, The Physiological Basis.* Bulletin of the World Health Organization Supplement to Vol. 67 (1989). Geneva: World Health Organization; 1991.

Andrusiak F, Larose-Kuzenko M. *The Effects of an Overactive Let-down Reflex.* Wayne, NJ: Avery Publishing Group; 1987: Lactation Consultant Series. Unit 13.

Aono T, Shioki T, Shoda T, Kurachi K. The initiation of human lactation and prolactin response to sucking. *J Clin Endocrinal Metab.* 1977;44:1101.

Aono T. Shioki T, Shoda T, et al. Studies in human lactation: milk composition and daily secretion rates of macronutrients in the first year of lactation. *Am J Clin Nutr.* 1991;54:69-80.

Auerbach, KG. Sequential and simultaneous breastpumping: a comparison. *Intl J Nurs Studies.* 1990;27:257-265.

Bohler E, Bergstrom S. Child growth during weaning depends on whether mother is pregnant again. *J Trop Pediatr.* Apr 1996;42(2):104-109.

Byrne, E. Breastmilk oversupply despite retained placental fragment. *J Hum Lact.* 1992;8(3):152.

Daly SEJ, Kent JC, Huynh DQ, et al. The determination of short-term volume changes and the rate of synthesis of human milk using computerized breast measurement. *Exp Physiol* 1992;77:79-87.

Day TW. Unilateral failure of lactation after breast biopsy. *J Fam Prac.* 1986;23(2):161-162.

De Carvalho M, Robertson S, Friedman A, et al. Effect of frequent breastfeeding on early milk production and infant weight gain. *Pediatrics.* 1983;72:307-311.

De Carvalho, M. et al. Effect of frequent breast-feeding on early milk production and infant weight gain. *Pediatrics.* 1983;72:307-311.

DeCoopman, Jan. Breastfeeding after pituitary resection: support for a theory of autocrine control of milk supply? *J Hum Lact.* 1993;9(1):35-40.

DelRe, RB et al. Prolactin inhibition and suppression of puerpural lactation by a Bf-ergocryptine (CB 154), a comparison with estrogen. *Obstet Gynecol.* 1973;41:884.

Dewey KG, Heinig MJ, Nommsen LA, Peerson JM, Lonnerdal B. Growth of breastfed and formula-fed infants from 0 to 18 months: the DARLING study. *Pediatrics.* 1992;89:1035-1041.

Hartmann, PE, Kulski, JK, Changes in the composition of the mammary secretion of women after abrupt termination of breastfeeding. *J Physiol (Lond).* 1977;74:509-510.

Healy DL, Rattigan S, Hartmann PE, et al. Prolactin in human milk: correlation with lactose, total protein and alpha-lactalbumin levels. *Am J Physiol.* 1980;238:E83-E86.

Hight-Laukaran V, Labbok MH, Peterson AE, Fletcher V, von Hertzen H, Van Look PF. Multicenter study of the Lactation Amenorrhea Method (LAM): II. Acceptability, utility, and policy implications. *Contraception.* June 1997;55(6):337-346.

Kennedy KI, Labbok MH, VanLook PFA. Consensus Statement: Lactational Amenorrhea Method for Family Planning. *Int J Obstet Gynecol.* 1996;(54):55-57.

Kippley S. *Breastfeeding and Natural Child Spacing.* New York: Harper & Row; 1989.

Klaus MH. The frequency of suckling-neglected but essential ingredient of breast-feeding. *Obstet Gynecol Clin North Am.* 1987;14:623-633.

Kulski JK, Hartmann PE. Changes in human milk composition during the initiation of lactation. *Austral J Exper Biol and Med Sci.* 1981;59:101-114.

Kurachi K. The initiation of human lactation and prolactin response to sucking. *J Clin Endocrinol Metab.* 1977;44:1101.

Labbok M, Cooney K, Coly S. *Guidelines: Breastfeeding, Family Planning, and the Lactational Amenorrhea Method (LAM).* Washington DC: Institute for Reproductive Health; 1994.

Labbok M, Krasovek K. Toward consistency in breastfeeding definitions. *Stud Fam Plan.* 1990;21(4):226-230.

Labbok MH, Hight-Laukaran V, Peterson AE, Fletcher V, von Hertzen H, Van Look PF. Multicenter study of the Lactation Amenorrhea Method (LAM): I. Efficacy, duration, and implications for clinical application. *Contraception.* June 1997; 55(6):327-336.

Matthews MK. The relationship between maternal labour analgesia and delay in the initiation of breastfeeding in healthy neonates in the early neonatal period. *Midwifery.* 1989;5:3-10.

Merchant K, Martorell R, Haas J. Maternal and fetal responses to the stresses of lactation concurrent with pregnancy and of short recuperative intervals. *Am J Clin Nutr.* 1990; 52(2):280-288.

Moscone SR, Moore MJ. Breastfeeding during pregnancy. *J Human Lact.* 1993;9(2):83-88.

Nagy GM, Arendt A, Banky Z, Halesz B. Dehydration attenuates plasma prolactin response to suckling through a dopaminergic mechanism. *Endocrinology.* 1992;130(2):819-824.

Neifert M, De Marzo S, Seacat S, Young P, Leff M, Orleans M. The influence of breast surgery, breast appearance, and pregnancy-induced breast changes on lactation sufficiency as measured by infant weight gain. *Birth.* Mar 1990; 17(1):31-38.

Neifert M. Breastfeeding after breast surgical procedure or breast cancer. *NAACOG's Clin Issues Perina Women's Health Nurs.* 1992;3(4):673-682.

Neifert M, McDonough SL, Neville MC. Failure of lactogenesis associated with placental retention. *Am J Obstet Gynecol.* 1981:140, 477-478.

Neifert M, Seacat JM, Jobe WE. Lactation failure due to insufficient glandular development. *Pediatrics.* 1985; 76:832-828.

Neville MC, Allen JC, Archer PC, et al. Studies in human lactation: milk volume and nutrient composition during weaning and lactogenesis. *Am J Clin Nutr.* 1991;54:81-92.

Neville MC, Neifert MR. *Lactation: Physiology, Nutrition, and Breastfeeding.* New York: Plenum Press; 1983.

Newman J. Breastfeeding problems associated with the early introduction of bottles and pacifiers. *J Human Lact.* 1990:6(2):59-63.

Newton MR, Newton N. Relation of the let-down reflex to the ability to breastfeed. *Pediatrics.* 1950;5:726.

Newton N. *Maternal Emotions.* New York: Paul E. Hoeber; 1955.

Newton N. Trebly sensuous woman. *Psych Today.* 1971;5:68-71, 98-99.

Perez A, Labbok MH, Queenan JT. Clinical study of the Lactational Amenorrhea Method for family planning. *Lancet.* Apr 18, 1992;339(8799): 968-970.

Reamer SB, Sugarman M. Breastfeeding beyond six months: mothers' perception of the positive and negative consequences. *J Trop Pediatr.* 1987; 33:93-97.

Riordan J, Rapp ET. Pleasure and purpose—the sensuousness of breastfeeding. *JOGN Nurs.* 1980;9:109-112.

Rodriguez-Garcia R, Frazier L. Cultural paradoxes relating to sexuality and breastfeeding. *J Human Lact* 1995;11(2):111-115.

Short RV, Lewis PR, Renfree MB, Shaw G. Contraceptive effects of extended Lactational Amenorrhea: beyond the Bellagio Consensus. *Lancet.* Mar 23, 1991;337(8743):715-717.

Slaven S, Harvey D. Unlimited suckling time improves breastfeeding. *Lancet.* 1983;1:392-393.

Spitz AM, Lee NC, Peterson HB. Treatment for lactation suppression: little progress in one hundred years. *Am J Obstet Gynecol.* Dec 1998;179(6): 1485-1490.

Stoppard M. *The Breast Book.* London: Dorling Kindersley Ltd; 1996.

Ueda T, Yokoyama Y, Irahara M, Aono T. Influence of psychological stress on suckling-induced pulsatile oxytocin release. *Obstet Gynecol.* 1994;84: 259-262.

Uvnas-Moberg K, Eriksson M. Breastfeeding: physiological, endocrine and behavourial adaptations causes by oxytocin and local neurogenic activity in the nipple and mammary gland. *Acta Paediat Scand.* 1996;85: 525-530.

Vekemans M. Postpartum contraception: the Lactational Amenorrhea Method. *Eur J Contracept Reprod Health Care.* June 1997;2(2):105-111.

Veronnen P. Breastfeeding—reasons for giving up and transient lactational crises. *Acta Paediatr Scand.* 1982;71:447-450.

Weber F, et al. An ultrasonographic study of the organization of sucking and swallowing by newborn infants. *Dev Med Child Neurol.* 1986;28:19-24.

Widstrom AM, Thingstrom-Paulsson J. The position of the tongue during rooting reflexes elicited in newborn infants before the first suckle. *Acta Paediatr Scand.* 1993;82:281-283.

Widstrom AM, Wahlberg V, et al. Short-term effects of early suckling and touch of the nipple on maternal behavior. *Early Hum Dev.* 1990; 21:153-163.

Woolridge M, et al. Individual patterns of milk intake during breastfeeding. *Early Hum Dev.* 1982;4:265-272.

Woolridge M. Anatomy of infant sucking. *Midwifery.* 1986;2:164-171.

Woolridge M, Baum JD. The regulation of human milk flow. In: Lindblad BS. *Perinatal Nutrition.* Vol 6. London: Academic Press; 1988.

Yamauchi Y, Yamanouchi I. Breastfeeding frequency during the first 24 hours after birth in fullterm neonates. *Pediatrics.* 1990;86(2):171-17.

3

Maternal and Infant Normal Nutrition and Biochemistry

In the exam blueprint, 10 to 16 questions are dedicated to maternal and infant normal nutrition and biochemistry, specifically: milk synthesis, diet, composition of milk, comparison between breastmilk and artificial feeding products/milks; ritual and traditional foods and introduction of other foods; maternal diet.

SUBTOPICS INCLUDED IN THIS CATEGORY

1. Definitions of breastfeeding (exclusive—partial—token)
2. Milk synthesis—compositional changes
3. Composition of milk
4. Comparison with artificial feeding products
5. Risks and hazards of other foods for infants
6. Ritual and traditional foods
   a. Introduction of foods other than human milk (the "what" of other foods)
   b. Cultural beliefs; inappropriate foods
7. Maternal diet and nutrition
   a. Normal weight gain and loss patterns
   b. Special diets; supplements
   c. Maternal ritual foods

CORE READING

_____. *The Womanly Art of Breastfeeding.* 6th rev ed. Schaumburg, IL: La Leche League International; 1997.

Bertelsen C, Auerbach KG. *Nutrition and Breastfeeding: The Cultural Connection.* Wayne, NJ: Avery Publishing Group; 1987: Lactation Consultant Series Unit 11.

Black RF, Jarman L, Simpson J. *Lactation Specialist Self-Study Modules #1-4.* Sudbury, MA: Jones & Bartlett Publishers; 1998: module 1 chap 2 A & B, module 3 chap 2A, module 4 chap 1C.

Institute of Medicine (Subcommittee on Nutrition during Lactation, Food and Nutrition Board). *Nutrition During Lactation.* Washington DC: National Academy of Sciences: 1991.

Kleinman RE, ed. *Pediatric Nutrition Handbook.* 4th ed. Elk Grove Village, IL: American Academy of Pediatrics; 1998.

Lauwers J, Shinskie D. *Counseling the Nursing Mother.* 3rd ed. Sudbury, MA: Jones & Bartlett Publishers; 2000: chaps 7, 8, 14, 16.

Lawrence RA. *Breastfeeding: a Guide for the Medical Profession,* 5th ed. St. Louis: Mosby; 1999: chaps 4, 7, 9, appendices A, B, C, I.

Morbacher N, Stock J. *The Breastfeeding Answer Book,* rev. ed. Schaumburg, IL: La Leche League International; 1997: chaps 6, 7, 8, 19.

Riordan J, Auerbach KG. *Breastfeeding and Human Lactation.* 2nd ed. Sudbury, MA: Jones & Bartlett Publishers; 1999: chaps 2, 5, 10, 15, appendix A.

Stuart-Macadam P, Dettwyler KA. *Breastfeeding: Biocultural Perspectives.* New York: Aldine De Gruyter; 1995: chaps 2, 3, 8.

Taylor MM. *Transcultural Aspects of Breastfeeding*—USA. Wayne, NJ: Avery Publishing Group; 1985: Lactation Consultant Series, Unit 2.

Worthington-Roberts B, Williams SR. *Nutrition in Pregnancy and Lactation.* 5th ed. St. Louis: Mosby; 1993.

ADDITIONAL RESOURCES

AAP and ACOG. *Guidelines for Perinatal Care.* 4th ed. Elk Grove Village, IL: American Academy of Pediatrics; 1997.

AAP workgroup on Breastfeeding. Breastfeeding and the Use of Human Milk. *Pediatrics.* 1997;100(6):1035-1039.

ADA. Position of the American Dietetic Association: Promotion of Breastfeeding. *J Am Diete Assoc.* 1997;97(6):662-666.

Akre J, ed. Infant Feeding, *The Physiological Basis.* Bulletin of the World Health Organization Supplement to Vol. 67 (1989). Geneva: World Health Organization; 1991.

Allen JC, Keller RP, Archer P, Neville MC. Studies in human lactation: milk composition and daily secretion rates of macronutrients in the first year of lactation. *Am J Clin Nutr.* 1991;54:69-80.

Anderson T, Foman SJ. Commercially prepared strained and junior foods for infants. *J Am Diet Assoc.* 1971;58.

Borwn KH, de Kanashirode HC, Del Aguila R, de Romana GL, Black RE. Milk consumption and hydration status of exclusively breastfed infants in a warm climate. *J Pediatr.* 1986; 108(1):677-680.

Casey CE, Neifert MR, Seacat JM, Neville MC. Nutrient intake by breastfed infants during the first five days after birth. *Am J Dis Child.* 1986; 140(9):933-936.

Dewey KG, Heinig J, Nommsen-Rivers L. Differences in morbidity between breastfed and formula-fed infants. *J Pediatr.* 1995;126:696-702.

Dewey KG, Heinig MJ, Nommsen LA, Lonnerdal B. Maternal versus infant factors related to breastmilk intake and residual milk volume: the DARLING study. *Pediatrics.* 1991;87(6):829-837.

Dewey KG, Heinig MJ, Nommsen LA, Peerson JM, Lonnerdal B. Breastfed infants are leaner than formula-fed infants at 1 y of age: the DARLING study. *Am J Clin Nutr.* 1993;57:140-145.

Dewey KG, Heinig MJ, Nommsen LA, Peerson JM, Lonnerdal B. Growth of breastfed and formula-fed infants from 0 to 18 months: the DARLING study. *Pediatrics.* 1992;89:1035-1041.

Diaz S, Herreros C, Aravena R, et al. Breastfeeding duration and growth of fully breastfed infants in a poor urban Chilean population. *Am J Clin Nutr.* 1995;62(2):371-376.

Fildes V. *Wet Nursing: a history from antiquity to the present.* New York: Basil Blackwell Ltd; 1988.

Foman SJ. *Nutrition of Normal Infants.* St. Louis: Mosby; 1993.

Fomon SJ, Filer LJ Jr, Anderson TA, Ziegler EE. Recommendations for feeding normal infants. *Pediatrics.* 1979;63(1):52-59.

Goldman AS, Garza C. Immunologic components in human milk during the second year of lactation. *Acta Paediatr Scand.* 1983;72:461-462.

Gulick E. The effects of breastfeeding on toddler health. *Pediatr Nurs.* 1986;12(1):51-4.

Heinig MH, Nommsen LA, Peerson MH, Lonnerdal B, Dewey KG. Energy and protein intakes of breastfed and formula-fed infants during the first year of life and their association with growth velocity: the DARLING study. *Am J Clin Nutr.* 1993;58:152-161.

Hendricks KM. Weaning recommendations: the scientific basis. *Nutr Rev.* 1992;50(5):125-133.

Hervada AR, Newman DR. Weaning: historical perspectives, practical recommendations, and current controversies. *Cur Prob Pediatr.* 1992;22(5):223-241.

Houston MJ, Howie PW, McNeilly AS. Factors affecting the duration of breastfeeding: 1. Measurement of breast milk intake in the first week of life. *Early Hum Dev.* 1983;8(1):49-54.

Howie PW, Houston MJ, Cook A, Smart L, McArdle T, McNeilly AS. How long should a breastfeed last? *Early Hum Dev.* 1981;5(1):71-77.

Imong SM, Jackson DA, Wongsawasdii L, et al. Predictors of breast milk intake in rural Thailand. *J Pediatr Gastroenterol Nutr.* 1989;8(3):359-370.

Institute of Medicine (Subcommittee on Nutrition during Lactation, Food and Nutrition Board). *Nutrition during Lactation.* Washington DC: National Academy of Sciences; 1991.

International Lactation Consultant Association: *Position Paper on Infant Feeding.* Raleigh, NC: ILCA; 1994.

Jensen R, ed. *Handbook of Milk Composition.* San Diego: Academic Press; 1995.

Jocson MA, Mason EO, Schanler RJ. The effects of nutrient fortification and varying storage conditions on host defense properties of human milk. *Pediatrics.* 1997;100:240-243.

Kulsoom U, Saeed A. Breastfeeding practices and beliefs about weaning among mothers of infants aged 0-12 months. *J Pak Med Assoc.* 1997; 47(2):54-60.

Kunz C, Lonnerdal B. Re-evaluation of the whey protein/casein ratio of human milk. *Acta Paediatr.* 1992;81(2):107-112.

Lonnerdal B, Forsum E. Casein content of human milk. *Am J Clin Nutr.* 1985;41(1):113-120.

Lucas A, Lucas PJ, Baum JD. Differences in the pattern of milk intake between breast and bottle fed infants. *Early Hum Dev.* 1981;5(2):195-199.

Lucas A, Lucas PJ, Baum JD. Pattern of milk flow in breastfed infants. *Lancet.* July 14, 1979;8133-8134.

Matheney RJ, Birch LL. Picciano MF. Control of intake by human-milk-fed infants: relationship between feeding size and interval. *Dev Psychobiol.* 1990;23(6):511-518.

Neifert MR. The optimization of breastfeeding in the perinatal period. *Clin Perinatol.* 1998;25(2):303-326.

Neville MC, Allen JC, Archer PC, Casey CE, et al. Studies in human lactation: milk volume and nutrient composition during weaning and lactogenesis. *Am J Clin Nutr.* 1991;54:81-92.

Neville MC, Allen JC, Archer PC, et al. Studies in human lactation: milk volume and nutrient composition during weaning and lactogenesis. *Am J Clin Nutr.* 1991;54:81-92.

Novello A. You can eat healthy & enjoy it. *Parade Magazine.* Nov. 11, 1990.

Paul K, Dittrichova J, Papousek H. Infant feeding behavior: development in patterns and motivation. *Devel Psychobiol.* 1996;29(7):563-576.

Raiha NC. Nutritional proteins in milk and the protein requirement of normal infants. *Pediatrics* 1985;1:136-141.

Sanchez-Hildago VM, Flores-Huerta S, Matute G, Serrano C, Urquieta B, Espinosa R. Whey protein/casein ratio and nonprotein nitrogen in preterm human milk during the first 10 days postpartum. *J Pediatr Gastroenterol Nutr.* 1998;26(1):64-69.

Satter E. *Child of Mine: Feeding with Love and Good Sense.* Palo Alto, CA: Bull Publishing; 1983.

Satter E. *How to Get Your Kid to Eat ... but Not too Much.* Palo Alto, CA: Bull Publishing, 1987.

Scammon RE, Doyle LO. Observations on the capacity of the stomach in the first ten days of postnatal life. *Am J Dis Child.* 1920;20:516-538.

Sievers E, Oldigs HD, Schultz-Lell G, Schaub J. Faecal excretion in infants. *Eur J Pediatr.* 1993;152(5):542-454.

Stuff JE, Nichols BL. Nutrient intake and growth performance of older infants fed human milk. *J Pediatr.* 1989;115:959-968.

Uvnas-Moberg K. The gastrointestinal tract in growth and reproduction. *Scientific American.* July 1989.

Weaver LT, Ewing G, Taylor LC. The bowel habit of milk-fed infants. *J Pediatr Gastroenterol Nutr.* Jul-Aug 1998;7(4):568-571.

Whitehead RG. The human weaning process. *Pediatrics* 1985;75(suppl): 189-193.

WHO/UNICEF: *Innocenti Declaration.* New York: UNICEF: 1990.

Wright P, MacLeod HA, Cooper MJ. Waking at night: the effect of early feeding experience. *Child Care Health Dev.* 1983;9(6):309-319.

Wright P. Learning experiences in feeding behaviour during infancy. *J Psychosom Res.* 1988;32(6):613-619.

Yamauchi Y, Yamanouchi I. Breastfeeding frequency during the first 24 hours after birth in full-term neonates. *Pediatrics.* 1990;86(2):171-175.

4

Maternal and Infant Immunology and Infectious Disease

In the exam blueprint, 11 to 19 questions are dedicated to maternal and infant immunology and infectious disease, specifically: antibodies; cross-infection; allergies/food sensitivity; and protection against infection.

SUBTOPICS INCLUDED IN THIS CATEGORY

1. Protection against infection
   a. Antibodies and protective factors in milk
   b. Immune systems
   c. Antiinflammatory properties
2. Cross-infection
   a. Bacteria and viruses in milk
   b. Maternal infections
   c. HIV and AIDS issues
3. Allergies/food sensitivities
   a. Etiologies; triggers
   b. Manifestations
   c. Management

CORE READING

Black RF, Jarman L, Simpson J. *Lactation Specialist Self-Study Modules #1-4.* Sudbury, MA: Jones & Bartlett Publishers; 1999: module 3 chap 2B.

Lauwers J, Shinskie D. *Counseling the Nursing Mother.* 3rd ed. Sudbury, MA: Jones & Bartlett Publishers; 2000: chaps 8, 11.

Lawrence RA, Lawrence RM. *Breastfeeding, a Guide for the Medical Profession.* 5th ed. St. Louis: Mosby; 1999: chaps 5, 16, 17, Appendix E.

Morbacher N, Stock J. *The Breastfeeding Answer Book.* rev. ed. Schaumburg, IL: La Leche League International; 1997: chap 23.

Rapp D. *Is This Your Child? Discovering and Treating Unrecognized Allergies in Children and Adults.* New York: Quill William Morrow; 1991.

Riordan J, Auerbach KG. *Breastfeeding and Human Lactation.* 2nd ed. Sudbury, MA: Jones & Bartlett Publishers; 1999: chap 5.

Lawrence R. *A Review of the Medical Benefits and Contraindications to Breastfeeding in the United States* (Maternal and Child Health Technical Information Bulletin). Arlington VA: National Center for Education in Maternal and Child Health; October 1997.

ADDITIONAL RESOURCES

Human Milk, Breastfeeding, and Transmission of Human Immunodeficiency Virus in the United States (RE9542). *Pediatrics.* 1995;96(5):977-979.

World Health Organization, UNICEF, and UNAIDS. *HIV and Infant Feeding: Infant Feeding Options.* Geneva: World Health Organization; 1998.

World Health Organization, UNICEF, and UNAIDS. *HIV and Infant Feeding: Guidelines for Decision-Makers.* Geneva: World Health Organization; 1998.

American Academy of Pediatrics, Committee on Pediatric AIDS. Human milk, breastfeeding, and transmission of human immunodeficiency virus in the United States. *Pediatrics.* 1995;96:977-979.

Bahna SL: Milk Allergy in Infancy. *Ann Allergy.* 1987;59:131-136.

Beaudry M, Dufour R, Marcoux S. Relation between infant feeding and infections during the first six months of life. *J Pediatr.* 1995;126:191-197.

Cant AJ, Marsden RA, Kilshaw PJ. Egg and cow's milk hypersensitivity in exclusively breastfed infants with eczema, and the detection of egg protein in breastmilk. *Br Med J.* 1985;291:982-935.

Cavataio F, Iacono G, Montalto G, et al. Clinical and pH-metric characteristics of gastroesophageal reflux secondary to cow's milk protein allergy. *Arch Dis Child.* 1996;75:51-56.

Centers for Disease Control and Prevention. Recommendations for assisting in the prevention of perinatal transmission of human T-lymphotropic virus type III/lymphadenopathy-associated virus and acquired immunodeficiency syndrome. *MMWR.* 1985;34:721-732.

Chandra RK, et al. Influence of maternal food antigen avoidance during pregnancy and lactation on incidence of atopic eczema in infants. *Clin Allergy.* 1986;16:563-569.

Chandra RK. Five-year follow-up of high-risk infants with family history of allergy who were exclusively breastfed or fed partial whey hydrolysate, soy, and conventional cow's milk formulas. *J Pediatr Gastroenterol Nutr.* 1997;24:380-388.

Chernishov VP, et al. Mucosal immunity of the mammary gland and immunology of mother/newborn interrelation. *Arch Immunol Ther Exp (Warsz).* 1990;38(1-2):145-164.

Clyne PS, Kulczycki A. Human breast milk contains bovine IgG. Relationship to infant colic? *Breastfeed Rev.* May 1992;218-222.

Coates MM, Riordan J. Breastfeeding during maternal or infant illness. *Clin Issues Perin Wom Health Nurs.* 1992;3:683-694.

Cochi SL, Fleming DW, Hightower AW, et al. Primary invasive *Haemophilus influenzae* type b disease: a population-based assessment of risk factors. *J Pediatr.* 1986;108:887-896.

Crook W. *Are You Allergic?* Jackson, TN: Professional Books; 1978.

Crook W. *Tracking Down Hidden Food Allergy.* Jackson, TN: Professional Books; 1980.

Crook W. *You and Allergy.* Jackson, TN: Professional Books; 1980.

Cunningham AS, Jelliffe DB, Jelliffe EFP. Breastfeeding and health in the 1980's: a global epidemiologic review. *J Pediatrics.* 1991;118(5):659-666.

Cunningham AS, Jelliffe DB, Jelliffe EFP. *Breastfeeding, Growth and Illness: an Annotated Bibliography.* New York: UNICEF; 1992.

De Boissieu D, et al. Multiple food allergy: a possible diagnosis in breastfed infants. *Acta Pediatr.* 1997;86:1042-1046.

Ellis MH, Short JA, Heiner DC. Anaphylaxis after ingestion of a recently introduced hydrolyzed whey protein formula. *J Pediatr.* 1991;118:74-77.

Falth-Magnusson K. Breast milk antibodies to foods in relation to maternal diet, maternal atopy and the development of atopic disease in the baby. *Int Arch Allergy Appl Immunol.* 1989;90(3):297-300.

Fishaut M, et al. Bronchomammary axis in the immune response to respiratory syncytial virus. *J Pediatr.* 1981;99(2):186-191.

Fukushima Y, et al. Consumption of cow milk and egg by lactating women and the presence of beta lactalbumin and ovalbumin in breastmilk. *Am J Clin Nutr.* 1997;65:30-35.

Garofalo R, et al. Interleukin-10 in human milk. *Pediatr Res.* 1995;37(4 Pt 1):444-449.

Garofalo RP, et al. Cytokines, chemokines, and colony-stimulating factors in human milk: the 1997 update. *Biol Neonate.* 1998;74(2):134-142.

Goldman AS, et al. Evolution of immunologic functions of the mammary gland and the postnatal development of immunity. *Pediatr Res.* 1998;43(2):155-162.

Goldman AS, et al. Host defenses: development and maternal contributions. *Adv Pediatr.* 1985;32:71-100.

Goldman AS, et al. Immunologic factors in human milk during the first year of lactation. *J Pediatr.* 1982;100(4):563-567.

Goldman AS, et al. Immunologic protection of the premature newborn by human milk. *Sem Perinatol.* 1994;18:495-501.

Goldman AS, et al. Transfer of maternal leukocytes to the infant by human milk. *Curr Top Microbiol Immunol.* 1997;222:205-213.

Goldman AS. Immunologic system in human milk. *J Pediatr Gastroenterol Nutr.* 1986;5(3):343-345.

Goldman AS. The immune system of human milk: antimicrobial, antiinflammatory and immunomodulating properties. *Pediatr Infect Dis J.* 1993;12(8):664-671.

Halken S, Host A, Hansen LG, et al. Effect of an allergy prevention programme on incidence of atopic symptoms in infancy. *Ann Allergy.* 1992;47:545-553.

Hanson LA, et al. Protective factors in milk and the development of the immune system. *Pediatrics.* 1985;75(1 Pt 2):172-176.

Hanson LA, et al. The immune response of the mammary gland and its significance for the neonate. *Ann Allergy.* 1984;53(6 Pt 2):576-582.

Hattevig G, et al. Affect of maternal avoidance of eggs, cow's milk and fish during lactation upon allergic manifestations in infants. *Clin Exp Allergy.* 1989;19:27-32.

Host A, Husby S, Osterballe O. A prospective study of cow's milk allergy in exclusively breastfed infants. *Acta Pediatr Scand.* 1988;77:663-670.

Howie PW, Forsyth JS, Ogston SA, Clark A, Florey C. Protective effect of breastfeeding against infection. *Br Med J.* 1990;300:11-16.

Huffman SL, Combest C. Role of breastfeeding in the prevention and treatment of diarrhea. *J Diar Dis Res.* 1990;8:68-81.

Iacono G, Carroccio A, Vatataio F, et al. Gastroesophageal reflux and cow's milk allergy in infants: a prospective study. *J Allergy Clin Immunol.* 1996;97:822-827.

Jakobsson I, Lindeberg T, Bemedoltsspm B, Jamsspm BG. Dietary bovine beta-lactoglobulin is transferred to human milk. *Acta Pediatr Scand.* 1985;74:342-345.

Jakobsson I, Lindeberg T. Cow's milk as a cause of infantile colic in breastfed infants. *Lancet.* 1978;2:437-439.

Jeliffe DB. Active anti-infective properties of human milk. *Lancet.* 1971; 2(7716):167-168.

Jensen RG. *Handbook of Milk Composition.* San Diego: Academic Press; 1995.

Kahn A. Mozin MJ, Rebuffat E, et al. Milk intolerance in children with persistent sleeplessness: a prospective double-blind crossover evaluation. *Pediatrics.* 1989;84(4):595-602.

Kajosaari M, et al. Prophylaxis of atopic disease by six months' total solid food elimination. Evaluation of 135 exclusively breast-fed infants of atopic families. *Acta Paediatr Scand.* 1983:72(3):411-4

Kleinman RE, ed. *Pediatric Nutrition Handbook.* 4th ed. Elk Grove Village, IL: American Academy of Pediatrics; 1998.

Lucas A, Brooke OG, Morley R, et al. Early diet of preterm infants and development of allergic or atopic disease: randomised prospective study. *Br Med J,* 1990;300:837-840.

Machida HM, Catto Smith AG, Gall DG, Travenen C, Scott RB. Allergic colitis in infancy: clinical and pathologic aspects. *J Pediatr Gastroenterol Nutr.* 1994;19:22-26.

Machtinger S, Moss R. Cow's milk allergy in breast-fed infants: the role of allergen and maternal secretory IgA antibody. *Allergy Clin Immunol.* 1986;77:341-347.

Meltzer EO. 100 of the best articles relevant to pediatric allergy and immunology: Synopsis book. *Pediatrics* 1990;85(5): Supplement.

Merrett TG, Burr ML, Butland BK, et al. Infant feeding and allergy: twelve-month prospective study of 500 babies in allergic families. *Ann Allergy* 1988;61(6 pt 2):13-20.

Mestecky J, ed. *Immunology of Milk and the Neonate.* New York: Plenum Press, 1991.

Newman J. How breast milk protects newborns. *Scientific American* Dec 1995;76-79.

Odze R, et al. Allergic colitis in infants. *J Pediatr.* 1995;126:163-170.

Odze RD, Wershil BK, Leichtner AM, Antonioli, DA. Allergic colitis in infants. *J Pediatr.* 1995;126:163-170.

Pooro E, et al. Early wheezing and breastfeeding. *J Asthma.* 1993;30(1): 23-28.

Popkin BM, Adair L, Akin JS, et al. Breast-feeding and diarrheal morbidity. *Pediatrics.* 1990;86:874-882.

Rapp D. *Is This Your Child? Discovering and Treating Unrecognized Allergies in Children and Adults.* New York: Quill William Morrow; 1991.

Rapp D. *Is This Your Child's World?* New York: Bantam Books; 1996.

Saarinen UM, Kajosaari M. Breastfeeding as prophylaxis against atopic disease: prospective follow-up study until 17 years old. *Lancet.* 1995;346: 1065-1069.

Saarinen UM. Prolonged breastfeeding as prophylaxis for recurrent otitis media. *Acta Paediatr Scand.* 1982;71:567-571.

Saylor JD, Bahna SL: Anaphylaxes to casein hydrolysate formula. *J Pediatr.* 1991;118:71-73.

Scariati PD, Grummer-Strawn LM, Fein SB. A Longitudinal analysis of infant morbidity and the extent of breastfeeding in the US. *Pediatrics.* 1997;99(6):e5.

Sigurs N, Hattevig G, Kjelman B. Maternal avoidance of eggs, cow's milk, and fish during lactation: effect on allergic manifestations, skin-prick tests, and specific IgE: Antibodies in children at age 4 years. *Pediatrics.* 1992;89:735-739.

Slade HB, Schwartz SA. Mucosal immunity: the immunology of breast milk. *J Allergy Clin Immunol.* 1987;80(3):348-356.

Steinman HA. "Hidden" allergens in foods. *J Allergy Clin Immunol.* 1996; 98(2):241-250.

Strimac JN, Chi DS. Significance of IgE level in amniotic fluid and cord blood for the prediction of allergy. *Ann Allergy.* 1986;61:133-136.

Strobel S. Dietary manipulation and induction of tolerance. *J Pediatr.* 1992; 121(5 pt 2):S74-79.

Wilson NW, Self TW, Hamburger RN. Severe cow's milk induced colitis. *Clin Pediatr.* 1990;29:77-80.

World Health Organization. Consensus statement from the consultation on HIV transmission and breastfeeding. *J Hum Lact.* 1992;8:173-174.

Wright AL, Holberg CJ, Martinez FR, Morgan WJ, Taussig LM. Breast-feeding and lower respiratory tract illness in the first year of life. *Br Med J.* 1989;299:946-949.

Wright AL, Holberg CJ, Taussig LM, Martinez FD. Relationship of infant feeding to recurrent wheezing at age 6 years. *Arch Pediatr Adolesc Med.* 1995;149:758-763.

Yap PL, et al. The development of mammary secretory immunity in the human newborn. *Acta Paediatr Scand.* 1981;70(4):459-465.

5 Maternal and Infant Pathology

In the exam blueprint, 19 to 33 questions are dedicated to maternal and infant pathology, specifically: acute/chronic abnormalities and diseases, both local and systemic; impact on lifelong health.

SUBTOPICS INCLUDED IN THIS CATEGORY

1. Acute illnesses and accidents—local and systemic
   a. Prematurity
      i. Milk issues—nutrition
      ii. Feeding issues
      iii. Management
   b. Birth-related
      i. Maternal—pregnancy complications; labor medications; Cesarean, placenta problems
      ii. Infant—adverse effects; early suck problems
   c. Acute illnesses and infections
      i. Engorgement, mastitis and breast infections
      ii. Infant or maternal infections including yeast
      iii. Jaundice; hypoglycemia
   d. Accidents
2. Chronic abnormalities and diseases—local & systemic
   a. Infant
      i. Genetic and metabolic
      ii. Neurologically impaired
      iii. Physical and structural; oral pathology
      iv. Gastrointestinal, digestive
   b. Maternal
      i. Chronic infections and conditions
      ii. Genetic and metabolic—e.g., diabetes, cancer

iii. Physical and sensory
iv. Breast problems

3. Impact on lifelong health—epidemiology of illnesses associated with feeding methods

CORE READING

Protecting, Promoting and Supporting Breastfeeding: The Special Role of Maternity Services. A Joint WHO/UNICEF statement. Geneva: World Health Organization Nutrition Unit; 1989.

Amir L, Hoover K, Mulford C. *Candidaisis and Breastfeeding.* Garden City Park, NJ: Avery Publishing Group; 1995: Lactation Consultant Series, Unit 18.

Black RF, Jarman L, Simpson J. *Lactation Specialist Self-Study Modules #1-4.* Sudbury, MA: Jones & Bartlett Publishers, 1999: module 2 chap 1A; 2B, C & D; module 4 chap 2 A & B, 3 A.

Danner S, Wilson-Clay B. *Breastfeeding the Infant with a Cleft Lip/Palate.* Wayne, NJ: Avery Publishing Group; 1986: Lactation Consultant Series, Unit 10.

Goer H. *Obstetric Myths Versus Research Realities: A Guide to the Medical Literature.* Westport, CT: Bergin & Garvey; 1995.

Korte D, Scaer R. *A Good Birth, a Safe Birth.* 3rd rev ed. Boston: The Harvard Common Press; 1992.

Lang S. *Breastfeeding Special Care Babies.* London: Balliere Tindall; 1997.

Lauwers J, Shinskie D. *Counseling the Nursing Mother.* 3rd ed. Sudbury, MA: Jones & Bartlett Publishers, 2000: chaps 12, 14, 16, 20, 12, 23.

Lawrence RA. *Breastfeeding, a Guide for the Medical Profession.* 5th ed. St. Louis: Mosby, 1999: chaps 8, 14, 15, 16, appendix B, appendix E.

Morbacher N, Stock J. *The Breastfeeding Answer Book.* rev ed. Schaumburg, IL: La Leche League International; 1997: chaps 11, 12, 13, 14, 20, 21, 22, 23.

Popper BK. *The Hospitalized Nursing Baby.* Schaumburg, IL: La Leche League International; 1998: Lactation Consultant Series II, Unit 1.

Riordan J, Auerbach KG. *Breastfeeding and Human Lactation.* 2nd ed. Sudbury, MA: Jones & Bartlett Publishers, 1999: chaps 7, 10, 11, 12, 13, 14, 15, 17, 20.

Royal College of Midwives. *Successful Breastfeeding.* 2nd ed. London: Churchill Livingstone; 1991.

Timko, SW, Culp YD, Pindell JG, Harakal R. *Breastfeeding the Baby with Down Syndrome.* Wayne, NJ: Avery Publishing Group; 1986: Lactation Consultant Series, Unit 9.

Walker M. *Breastfeeding Premature Babies.* Wayne, NJ: Avery Publishing Group; 1990: Lactation Consultant Series, Unit 14.

Walker M. *Mastitis in Lactating Women.* Schaumburg IL: La Leche League International; 1999: Lactation Consultant Series II, Unit 2.

Wolf LS, Glass RP. *Feeding And Swallowing Disorders In Infancy.* Tucson, AZ: Therapy Skill Builders; 1992.

Engelking C, Page-Lieberman J. *Maternal Diabetes and Diabetes in Young Children: Their Relationship to Breastfeeding.* Wayne, NJ: Avery Publishing Group; 1986: Lactation Consultant Series, Unit 5.

ADDITIONAL RESOURCES

_____. Mastitis. *Lippincotts Prim Care Pract.* Mar-Apr 1998; 2(2):184-148.

_____. *The Mother-Friendly Childbirth Initiative.* Washington DC: Coalition for Improving Maternity Services; 1996.

Alexander JM, Grant AM, Campbell MJ. Randomized controlled trial of breast shells and Hoffman's exercises for inverted and non-protractile nipples. *Br Med J.* 1992;304:1030-1032.

Als H, Lester BM, Tronick E, Brazelton TB. Manual for the assessment of preterm infants' behavior (AFPB). In Fitzgerald JE, Lester BM, Jogman MW, eds. *Theory and Research in Behavioral Pediatrics.* Vol, 1. New York: Plenum; 1982:64-133.

Amir L, Hoover K, Mulford C. *Candidiasis & Breastfeeding.* Wayne, NJ: Avery Publishing Group, 1995; Lactation Consultant Series, Unit 18.

Amir L. Eczema of the nipple and breast: a case report. *J Hum Lact.* Sep 1993;9(3):173-175.

Amir LH, Dennerstein L, Garland SM, Fisher J, Farish SJ. Psychological aspects of pain in lactating women. *J Psychosom Obstet Gynaecol.* Mar 1996; 17(1):53-58.

Amir LH, Garland SM, Dennerstein L, Farish SJ. *Candida albicans:* is it associated with nipple pain in lactating women? *Gynecol Obstet Invest.* 1996;41(1):30-34.

Amir LH, Pakula S. Nipple pain, mastalgia and candidiasis in the lactating breast. *Aust N Z J Obstet Gynaecol.* Nov 1991; 31(4):378-380.

Amir LH. Candida and the lactating breast; predisposing factors. *J Hum Lact.* Dec 1991;7(4):177-181.

Anderson GC. Risk in mother-infant separation post birth. *Image: J Nurs Scholarship.* Winter 1989;21(4):196-199.

Andrusiak F, Larose-Kuzenko M. *The Effects of an Overactive Let-down Reflex.* Wayne NJ: Avery Publishing Group; 1987: Lactation Consultant Series, Unit 13.

Ardran GM, et al. A cineradiographic study of breastfeeding. *Br J Radiol* 1958;31(363):156-162.

Arsenault G. Using a disposable syringe to treat inverted nipples. *Can Fam Physician* Sep 1997;43:1517-1518.

Auerbach KG, Gartner LM. Breastfeeding and human milk: their association with jaundice in the neonate. *Clin Perinatol.* 1987;14:89-107.

Bahna SL: Milk allergy in infancy. *Ann Allergy.* 1987;59:131-136.

Bergman DA, ed. *Practice Parameters from the American Academy of Pediatrics: a Compilation of Evidence-based Guidelines for Pediatric Practice.* Elk Grove Village, IL: American Academy of Pediatrics; 1997.

Bosque EM, et al. Physiologic measures of kangaroo vs. incubator care in a tertiary-level nursery. *JOGNN.* 24:210-26.

Brown KH. Dietary management of acute childhood diarrhea: optimal timing of feeding and appropriate use of milks and mixed diets. *J Pediatr.* 1991;118:S92-98.

Brown LP, et al. Incidence and pattern of jaundice in healthy breastfed infants during the first month of life. *Nurs Res.* 1993;42:108-110.

Buchko BL, Pugh LC, Bishop BA, Cochran JF, Smith LR, Lerew DJ. Comfort measures in breastfeeding, primiparous women. *JOGNN.* Jan 1994; 23(1):46-52.

Burke Snyder J. *Variations in Infant Palatal Structure.* [master's thesis]. Iowa: Joanne Burke Snyder; 1996.

Byrne, E. Breastmilk oversupply despite retained placental fragment. *J Hum Lact.* 1992;8(3):152.

Cable B, Stewart M, Davis J. Nipple wound care: a new approach to an old problem. *J Hum Lact.* Dec 1997;13(4):313-318.

Chen DC, et al. Stress during labor and delivery and early lactation performance. *Am J. Clin Nutr.* 1998;68(2):335-344.

Coates MM, Riordan J. Breastfeeding during maternal or infant illness. *Clin Issues Perin Wom Health Nurs.* 1992;3:683-694.

Coates, MM. Nipple pain related to vasospasm in the nipple? *J Hum Lact.* 1992;8(3):153.

Combs VL, Marino BL. A comparison of growth patterns in breast and bottle-fed infants with congenital heart disease. *Pediatr Nurs.* 1993;19: 175-179.

Cristensson K, Siles C, Moreno L et al. Temperature, metabolic adaption and crying in healthy full-term newborns cared for skin-to-skin or in a cot. *Acta Pediatr.* 1992;81:488-493.

Crowell MK, Hill PD, Humenick, SS. Relationship between obstetric analgesia and time of effective breastfeeding. *Nurse-Midwifery.* 1994;39(3): 150-156.

Dahlen H. Lactation mastitis. *Nurs Times.* 1993;89(36):38-40.

Dahm LS, James LS: Newborn temperature and calculated heat loss in the delivery room. *Pediatrics.* 1972;49:504.

De Boissieu D, et al. Multiple food allergy: a possible diagnosis in breastfed infants. *Acta Pediatr.* 1997;86:1042-1046.

De Carvalho M, Hall M, Harvey D. Effects of water supplementation on physiological jaundice in breastfed babies. *Arch Dis Child.* 1981; 569-569.

De Carvalho M, Klaus MH, Merkatz RB. Frequency of breast-feeding and serum bilirubin concentration. *Am J Dis Child.* 1982;136:737-738.

De Carvalho M, Robertson S, Friedman A, et al. Effect of frequent breast-feeding on early milk production and infant weight gain. *Pediatrics.* 1983;72:307-311.

De Carvalho M, Robertson S, Klaus M. Fecal bilirubin excretion and serum bilirubin concentrations in breastfed and bottle-fed infants. *J Pediatr.* 1985;107:786-790.

Dixon JM, Ravisekar O, Chetty U, Anderson TJ. Periductal mastitis and duct ectasia: different conditions with different aetiologies. *Br J Surg.* 1996;83(6):820-822.

Dodd KL. Neonatal jaundice: a lighter touch. *Arch Dis Child.* 1993;68: 529-532.

Duffy EP, Percival P, Kershaw E. Positive effects of an antenatal group teaching on postnatal nipple pain, nipple trauma and breastfeeding rates. *Midwifery.* 1997;13(4):189-196.

Duncan LL, Elder SB. Breastfeeding the infant with PKU. *J Hum Lact.* 1997;13:231-235.

Eidelman, Al, Hoffmann NW, Kaitz M: Cognitive deficits in women after childbirth. *Obstet Gynecol.* 1993;81:764-767.

Evans K, Evans R, Simmer K. Effect of method of breastfeeding on breast engorgement, mastitis, and infantile colic. *Acta Pediatr.* 1995;84(8): 849-852.

Fetherston C. Characteristics of lactation mastitis in a Western Australia cohort. *Breastfeed Rev.* 1997;5(2):5-11.

Fetherston C. Risk factors for lactation mastitis. *J Hum Lact.* 1998; 14(2):101-109.

Fisher C. A midwife's view of the history of modern breastfeeding practices. *Int J Gynaecol Obstet.* 1990; 31(suppl 1):47-50, discussion 67-68.

Ford RPK, Taylor BJ, Mitchell EA, et al. Breastfeeding and the risk of sudden infant death syndrome. *Int J Epidemiol.* 1993;22:885-890.

Foxman B, Schwartz K, Looman SJ. Breastfeeding practices and lactation mastitis. *Soc Sci Med.* Mar 1994;38(5):755-761.

Frank D. Sore nipples. *J Obstet Gynecol Neonatal Nurs.* Nov-Dec 1997; 26(6):629-630.

Franklin R, O'Grady C, Carpenter L. Neonatal thyroid function: comparison between breastfed and bottle-fed infants. *J Pediatr.* 1985;106:124-126.

Frantz KB. *Breastfeeding Product Guide.* Sunland, CA. Geddes Productions; 1993.

Fraval MMPR. A pilot study: osteopathic treatment of infants with a sucking dysfunction. *AAO J.* 1998;8(2):25-33.

Fusi L, Maresh JJA, Steer PJ, Beard RW. Maternal pyrexia associated with the use of epidural analgesia in labor. *Lancet.* 1989;(1):1250-1252.

Gartner LM, Auerbach KG. Breast milk and breastfeeding jaundice. *Adv Pediatr.* 1987;34:249-274.

Gartner LM. Introduction. Gartner LM, ed. Breastfeeding in the hospital. *Semin Perinatol.* 1994;18:475.

Gartner LM. Management of jaundice in the well baby. *Pediatrics* 1992; 89:826-827.

Gartner LM. Neonatal jaundice. *Pediatr Rev.* 1994;15:422-432.

Greve L, et al. Breastfeeding in the management of the newborn with phenylketonuria: a practical approach to dietary therapy. *J Am Diet Assoc.* 1994;94:305-309.

Habbick BF, Khanna C, To T. Infantile hypertrophic pyloric stenosis: a study of feeding practices and other possible causes. *Can Med Assoc J.* 1989;104:401-404.

Hahn HB, et al. Breastfeeding and neonatal screening for congenital hypothyroidism. *Tex Med.* 1986;82:46-47.

Hamosh M. Digestion in the premature infant: the effects of human milk. *Sem Perinatol.* 1994;18:485-494.

Hancock KE, Spangler AK. There's a fungus among us! *J Hum Lact.* 1993;9(3):179-180.

Hattevig G, et al. Affect of maternal avoidance of eggs, cow's milk and fish during lactation upon allergic manifestations in infants. *Clin Exp Allergy.* 1989;19:27-32.

Heacock HJ, et al. Influence of breast vs. formula milk on physiological gastroesophageal reflux in healthy newborn infants. *J Pediatr Gastroenterol Nutr.* 1992;14:41-46.

Heads J. Too much emphasis on nipple creams. *J Hum Lact.* Dec 1997; 13(4):274-275.

Hill PD, Hanson KS, Mefford AL. Mothers of low birthweight infants: breastfeeding patterns and problems. *J Hum Lact.* 1994;10:169-176.

Hill P, Humenick S. The occurrence of breast engorgement. *J Hum Lact.* 1994;10(2):79-86.

Hoffman, JB. A suggested treatment for inverted nipples. *Am J Obstet Gynecol.* 1953;66:346.

Hogan C. Mastitis and breastfeeding. *Aust Fam Physician.* Jan 1994; 23(1):77.

Holiday KE, et al. Growth of human milk-fed and formula fed infants with cystic fibrosis. *J Pediatr Gastroenterol Nutr.* 1991;118:77-79.

Hopkinson J. Interfeeding breast pain: a case report. *J Hum Lact.* Sep 1992;8(3):149-151.

Host A, Husby S, Osterballe O. A prospective study of cow's milk allergy in exclusively breastfed infants. *Acta Pediatr Scand.* 1988;77:663-670.

Howie PW, Forsyth JS, Ogston SA, Clark A, Florey C. Protective effect of breastfeeding against infection. *Br Med J.* 1990;300:11-16.

Howie PW, Houston MJ, Cook A, Smart L, McArdle T, McNeilly AS. How long should a breast feed last? *Early Hum Dev.* 1981;5(1):71-77.

Huffman SL, Combest C. Role of breastfeeding in the prevention and treatment of diarrhea. *J Diar Dis Res.* 1990;8:68-81.

Huggins KE, Billon SF. Twenty cases of persistent sore nipples: collaboration between lactation consultant and dermatologist. *J Hum Lact.* Sep 1993;9(3):155-160.

Humenick SS, Hill PD, Anderson MA. Breast engorgement: patterns and selected outcomes. *J Hum Lact.* 1994;10:897-93.

Huml SC. Moist wound healing for cracked nipples in the breastfeeding mother. *Leaven.* Jan-Feb 1994:3-6.

Hunziker UA and Barr RG. Increased carrying reduces infant crying: a randomized controlled trial. *Pediatrics.* 1986;77:641-647.

Inch S, Renfew MJ. Common breastfeeding problems. In: *Effective care in Pregnancy and Childbirth.* Oxford: Oxford University Press; 1989.

Inch S, Fisher C. Mastitis: infection or inflammation? *Practitioner.* Aug 1995;239(1553):472-476.

Inch S. Antenatal preparation for breastfeeding. In: *Effective Care in Pregnancy and Childbirth,* Vol 1. Pregnancy. Oxford: Oxford University Press; 1989.

Inoue N, Sakashita R, Kamegai T. Reduction of masseter muscle activity in bottle-fed babies. *Early Hum Dev* 1995;42:185-193.

Ironside JW, Guthrie W. The galactocele: a light- and electronmicroscopic study. *Histopathology.* 1985;9:457-467.

Jakobsson I, Lindeberg T. Cow's milk as a cause of infantile colic in breast-fed infants. *Lancet.* 1978;2:437-439.

Johnstone HA, Marcinak JF. Candidiasis in the breastfeeding mother and infant. *J Obstet Gynecol Neonatal Nurs.* Mar-Apr 1990;19(2):171-173.

Kaufmann R, Foxman B. Mastitis among lactating women: occurrence and risk factors. *Soc Sci Med.* 1991;33(6):701-705.

Kessaree N. Treatment of inverted nipples using a disposable syringe. *Indian Pediatr.* Mar 1993;30(3):429-430.

Kinlay JR, et al. Incidence of mastitis in breastfeeding women during the six months after delivery: a prospective cohort study. *Med J Aust.* Sep 21 1998;169(6):310-312.

Kostraba JH, Cruickshanks KJ, et al. Early exposure to cow's milk and solid foods in infancy, genetic predisposition, and risk of IDDM. *Diabetes.* 1993;42:288-295.

Kron RE, Stein M, Goddard KE: Newborn sucking behavior affected by obstetric sedation. *Pediatrics.* 1966;37:1012-1016.

Kuhnert B. Obstetric medication and neonatal behavior: current controversies. *Clin Perinatal.* June 1985;12:423-440.

L'Esperance C, Franz K. Time limitation for early breastfeeding. *J Obstet Gynecol Neonatal Nurs.* Mar-Apr 1985;14(2):1114-1148.

La Vergne NA. Does application of tea bags to sore nipples while breastfeeding provide effective relief? *J Obstet Gynecol Neonatal Nurs.* Jan-Feb 1997;26(1):53-58.

Labbok MH, Colie C. Puerperium and breast-feeding. *Curr Opin Obstet Gynecol.* 1992;4:818-825.

Labbok MH, Hendershot BD. Does breastfeeding protect against malocclusion? An analysis of the 1981 child health supplement to the National Health Interview Survey. *Am J Prev Med.* 1987;3:227-232.

Lawlor-Smith L, Lawlor-Smith C. Vasospasm—a manifestation of Raynaud's phenomenon: case reports. *BMJ.* Mar 1 1997;314(7081):644-645.

Lawlor-Smith LS. Lawlor-Smith CL. Raynaud's phenomenon of the nipple: a preventable cause of breastfeeding failure? *Med J Aust.* Apr 21 1997; 166(8):448.

Livingstone V. Breastfeeding kinetics: A problem solving approach to breastfeeding difficulties. *World Rev Nutr Diet.* 1995;78:28-54.

Livingstone VH, Willis CE, Berkowitz J. Staphylococcus aureus and sore nipples. *Can Fam Physician.* Apr 1996;42:654-659.

Lombardino LJ, Stapell JB, Gerhardt KJ. Evaluating communicative behaviors in infancy. *J Pediat Healthcare.* 1987;1(5):240-246.

Loon JL, Humenick SS. Breast engorgement: contributing variables and variables amenable to nursing intervention. *J Obstet Gynecol Neonatal Nurs.* Jul-Aug 1989;18(4):309-315.

Lopez-Alarcon J, Villapando S, Fajardo A. Breastfeeding lowers the frequency and duration of acute respiratory infection and diarrhea in infants under six months of age. *J Nutr.* 1997;127:436-443.

Lucas A, Cole T. Breastmilk and neonatal necrotizing enterocolitis. *Lancet.* 1990;339:261-264.

Lucas A, et al. A randomized multicentre study of human milk versus formula and later development in preterm infants. *Arch Dis Child.* 1994; 70:F140-146.

Lucas A, et al. Breastmilk and subesquent intelligence quotient in children born preterm. *Lancet.* 1992;339:261-264.

Lucas A, et al. Early diet in preterm infants and developmental status at 18 months. *Lancet.* 1990b;335:1477-1481.

Lucas A, et al. Randomized outcome trial of human milk fortification and developmental outcome in preterm infants. *Am J Clin Nutr.* 1996;64: 142-151.

Luder E, et al. Current recommendations for breastfeeding in cystic fibrosis centers. *Am J Public Health.* 1992;82:1380-1382.

MacArthur C, Letis M, Knox EG. Investigation of long term problems after obstetric epidural anesthesia. *B Med J.* 1992;304:1279-1282.

Macdonald H. Candida: the hidden deterrent to breastfeeding. *Can Nurse.* 1995;91(9):27-30.

Maher, SM. An overview of solutions to breastfeeding and sucking problems. La Leche League International; 1988. Schaumburg, IL.

Maisels MJ, et al. Jaundice in the healthy newborn infant: a new approach to an old problem. *Pediatrics.* 1988;81:505-511.

Maisels MJ, et al. The effect of breastfeeding frequency on serum bilirubin levels. *Am J Obstet Gynecol.* 1994;170:880-883.

Maisels MJ, Gifford K. Neonatal jaundice in full term infants: role of breastfeeding and other causes. *Am J Dis Child.* 1983;137:561-562.

Maisels MJ, Newman TB. Kernicterus in otherwise healthy, breastfed term newborns. *Pediatrics.* 1995;96:730-733.

Marmet C, Shell E. Training neonates to suck correctly. *Am J Maternal Child Nurs.* 1984;9:401-407.

Marshall BR, Hepper JK, Zirbel CC. Sporadic puerperal mastitis. An infection that need not interrupt lactation. *JAMA.* 1975; 233(13):1377-1379.

Marshall DR, Callan PP, Nicholson W. Breastfeeding after reduction mammaplasty. *Br J Plast Surg.* 1994;47(3):167-169.

Martinez JC, et al. Hyperbilirubinemia in the breastfed newborn: a controlled trial of four interventions. *Pediatrics.* 1993;91:470-473.

Mathew OP, Bhatia J. Sucking and breathing patterns during breast- and bottle-feeding in term neonates. *AJDC.* 1989;143:588-592.

Mathew, OP. Science of bottle feeding. *Pediatrics.* 1991;119(4):511-519.

Matthews MK. The relationship between maternal labour analgesia and delay in the initiation of breastfeeding in healthy neonates in the early neonatal period. *Midwifery.* 1989;5:3-10.

McBride MC, Danner SC. Sucking disorders in neurologically impaired infants: assessment and facilitation of breastfeeding. *Clin Perinatol.* 1987; 14:109-130.

McCabe L, et al. The management of breastfeeding among infants with phenylketonuria. *J Inherit Metal Dis.* 1989;12:467-474.

McClure VS. *Infant Massage: A Handbook for Loving Parents.* New York: Bantam Books; 1989.

McGeorge DD. The "Niplette": an instrument for the non-surgical correction of inverted nipples. Br J Plast Surg. 1994;47(1):46-49.

Mehta A. Prevention in management of neonatal hypoglycemia. *Arch Dis Child.* 1994;70:F54-F65.

Meier P. Bottle- and breastfeeding: effects on transcutaneous oxygen pressure and temperature in preterm infants. *Nurs Res.* 1988;37(1):36-41.

Meier PP, Brown LP. State of the science: breastfeeding for mothers and low birth weight infants. *Nurs Clin North Am.* 1996;31:351-365.

Meier PP, et al. Breastfeeding support services in the neonatal intensive care unit. *JOGNN.* 1993;22:338-344.

Meier PP. Bottle and breastfeeding: effects on transcutaneous oxygen pressure and temperature in preterm infants. *Nurs Res.* 1988;37:36-41.

Melnikow J, Bedinghaus JM. Management of common breastfeeding problems. *J Fam Pract.* 1994; 39(1):56-64.

Minchin M, Minogue C, Meehan M, et al. Expanding the WHO/UNICEF Baby Friendly Hospital Initiative (BFHI): Eleven Steps to optimal infant feeding in a pediatric unit. *Breastfeeding Rev.* 1996;4:87-91.

Minchin MK. Positioning for breastfeeding. *Birth.* 1989;16(2):67-73; discussion 74-80.

Misulta H, et al. Thyroid hormones in human milk and their influence on thyroid function of breastfed babies. *Pediatr Res.* 1983;17:4068.

Mitchell EA, Stewart MW, Becroft DM, et al. Results from the first year of the New Zealand cot death study. *NZ Med J.* 1991;104:71-76.

Mitchell EA, Taylor BJ, Ford RPK, et al. Four modifiable and other major risk factors for cot death: the New Zealand study. *J Paediatr Child Health.* 1992;28:S3-S8.

Moon JL, Humenick SS. Breast engorgement: contributing variables and variables amenable to nursing intervention. *J Obstet Gynecol Neonatal Nurs.* Jul-Aug 1989;18(4):309-315.

Narayanan I. Sucking on the "emptied" breast—a better method of non-nutritive sucking than use of a pacifier. *Ind Pediatr.* 1990;27:1122-1123.

Neifert M, De Marzo S, Seacat S, Young P, Leff M, Orleans M. The influence of breast surgery, breast appearance, and pregnancy-induced breast changes on lactation sufficiency as measured by infant weight gain. *Birth.* 1990;17(1):31-38.

Neifert M, Seacat J. Practical aspects of breastfeeding the premature infant. *Perin Neonatol.* 1988;12:24-30.

Neifert, M. Breastfeeding after breast surgical procedure or breast cancer. *NAACOG's Clin Issues Perinat Women's Health Nurs.* 1992;3(4):673-682.

Neifert M, McDonough SL, Neville, MC. Failure of lactogenesis associated with placental retention. *Am J Obstet Gynecol.* 1981;140:477-478.

Neifert M, Seacat JM, Jobe WE. Lactation failure due to insufficient glandular development. *Pediatrics.* 1985;76:832-828.

Newman J. Breastfeeding problems presenting to the emergency department: diagnosis and management. Pediatr Emerg Care. 1989;5(3):198-201.

Newman TB, Maisels MJ. Evaluation and treatment of jaundice in the term newborn: a kinder, gentler approach. *Pediatrics.* 1992;89:809-818.

Newman, Jack. Breastfeeding problems associated with the early introduction of bottles and pacifiers. *J Hum Lact.* 1990;6(2):59-63.

Newton MR and Newton N. Relation of the let-down reflex to the ability to breastfeed. *Pediatrics.* 1950;5:726.

Nicodem VC, Danziger D, Gebka N, et al. Do cabbage leaves prevent breast engorgement? A randomized, controlled study. *Birth.* 1993;20:61-64.

Odze R, et al. Allergic colitis in infants. *J Pediatr.* 1995;126:163-170.

Ogle KS, Davis S. Mastitis in lactating women. *J Fam Prac.* 1988;26(2):139-144.

Palmer MM. *The Normal Acquisition of Oral Feeding Skills; Implications for Assessment and Treatment.* New York: Theraputic Media; 1982.

Papaefthymiou G, Oberhauer R, Pendl G. Craniocerebral birth trauma caused by vacuum extraction: a case of growing skull fracture as a perinatal complication. *Childs Nervous Syst.* 1996;12(2):117-120.

Paradise JL, et al. Evidence in infants with cleft palate that breastmilk protects against otitis media. *Pediatrics.* 1994;94:853-860.

Polberger S, Lonnerdal B. Simple and rapid macronutrient analysis in human milk for individualized fortification: basis for improved nutritional management of very-low birthweight infants? *J Pediatr Gastroenterol Nutr.* 1993;17:283-290.

Pugh LC, Buchko BL, Bishop BA, Cochran JF, Smith LR, Lerew DJ. A comparison of topical agents to relieve nipple pain and enhance breastfeeding. *Birth.* 1996;23(2):88-93.

Rench MA, Baker CJ. Group B streptococcal breast abscess in a mother and mastitis in her infant. *Obstet Gynecol.* 1989;73(5 pt 2):875-877.

Reynolds JL. Post-traumatic stress disorder after childbirth: the phenomenon of traumatic birth. *CMAJ.* 1997;156(6):831-835.

Righard L, Alade MO. Sucking technique and its effect on success of breastfeeding. *Birth.* 1992;19(4):185-189.

Righard L, Alade, MO. Effect of delivery room routines on success of first breast-feed. *Lancet.* 1990;336:1105-1107.

Righard L. Are breastfeeding problems related to incorrect breastfeeding technique and the use of pacifiers and bottles? *Birth.* 1998;25(1): 40-44.

Riordan JM, et al. A descriptive study of lactation mastitis in long-term breastfeeding women. *J Hum Lact.* 1990;6(2):53-58.

Riva E. et al. Early breastfeeding is linked to higher intelligence quotient scores in dietary treated phenylketonuric children. *Acta Pediatr.* 1996;85: 56-58.

Roberts KL, Reiter M, Schuster D. Effects of cabbage leaf extract on breast engorgement. *J Hum Lact.* 1998;14(3):231-236.

Roberts KL, Retier M, Schuster D. A comparison of chilled and room temperature cabbage leaves in treating breast engorgement. *J Hum Lact.* 1995;11:191-194.

Roberts KL: A comparison of chilled cabbage leaves and chilled gelpaks in reducing breast engorgement. *J Hum Lact.* 1995;11:17-20.

Rogan WJ, Gladen BC. Breastfeeding and cognitive development. *Early Human Dev.* 1993;31:181-193.

Rosier W. Cool cabbage compresses. *Breastfeed Rev.* 1988;28-31.

Ross MW. *Back to the Breast: Retraining Infant Suckling Patterns.* Wayne, NJ: Avery Publishing Group; 1987: Lactation Consultant Series, Unit 15.

Rovet JF. Does breastfeeding protect the hypothyroid infant whose condition is diagnosed by newborn screening. *Am J Dis Child.* 1990;144: 319-323.

Russell R, et al. Assessing long term backache after childbirth. *BMJ.* 1993;306:1299-1303.

Sassen ML, Brand R, Grote JJ. Breastfeeding and acute otitis media. *Am J Otolaryngol.* 1994;15:351-357.

Scanlon JW, Ostheimer GW, et al. Neurobehavioral responses and drug concentrations in newborns after maternal epidural anesthesia with bupivicaine. *Anesthesiology.* 1976;45:400-405.

Schanler RJ. Suitablity of human milk for the low birthweight infant. *Clin Perinatol.* 1995;22:207-222.

Sepkoski CM, Lester BM, Ostheimer GW, Brazelton TB. The effect of maternal epidural anesthesia on neonatal behavior during the first month. *Dev Med Child Neurol.* 1992;34:1072-1080.

Sexson WR. Incidence of neonatal hypoglycemia: a matter of definition. *J Pediatr.* 1984;105:149-150.

Shrago L, Bocar D. The infant's contribution to breastfeeding. *JOGNN.* 1990;19(3):209-215.

Slaven S, Harvey D. Unlimited suckling time improves breastfeeding. *Lancet.* 1983;1:392-393.

Smith W, et al. Physiology of sucking in the normal term infant using real-time ultrasound. *Radiology* 1985;156:379.

Snyder JD, Rosenblum N, Wershil B, Goldman H, Winter HS. Plyoric stenosis and eosinophilic gastroenteritis in infants. *J Pediatr Gastroenterol Nutr.* 1987;6:543-547.

Sosa R, Kennell JH, Klaus M, et al. The effect of early mother-infant contact on breast feeding, infection and growth. In: Lloyd JK, ed. *Breastfeeding and the Mother.* Amsterdam: Elsevier; 1976:179-193.

Spitz AM, Lee NC, Peterson HB. Treatment for lactation supression: little progress in one hundred years. *Am J of Obstet and Gynecol.* 1998;179(6): 1485-1490.

Stine LH. Breastfeeding the premature newborn: a protocol without bottles. *J Hum Lact.* 1990;6:167-170.

Stoppard M. *The Breast Book.* London: Dorling Kindersley Ltd; 1996.

Swift K. Non-nursing mothers' use of active breast binding vs. passive 24-hour support bra wearing: a comparative study. [unpublished master's thesis]. Louisiana State University.

Tanguay KE, McBean MR, Jain E. Nipple candidiasis among breastfeeding mothers. Case-control study of predisposing factors. *Can Fam Physician.* 1994;40:1407-1413.

Tanoue Y, Oda S. Weaning time of children with infantile autism. *J Autism Dev Disord.* 1989;19(3):425-434.

Terrill PJ, Stapleton MJ. The inverted nipple: to cut the ducts or not? *Br J Plast Surg.* Jul 1991;44(5):372-377.

Theberge-Rousselet D. The treatment of mastitis in nursing mothers. *Can Nurse.* 1976;72(3):32.

Thomassen P, Johansson VA, Wassberg C, Petrini B. Breastfeeding, pain and infection. *Gynecol Obstet Invest.* 1998;46(2):73-74.

Thorley V. Inverted nipple with fatty plaques on areola and nipple. *Breastfeed Rev.* 1997;5(2):43-44.

Timko SW, Culp YD, Pindell JG, Harakal R. *Breastfeeding the Baby with Down Syndrome.* Wayne, NJ: Avery Publishing Group; 1986: Lactation Consultant Series, Unit 9.

Tronick E, Wise S, Brazelton TB, et al. Regional obstetric anesthesia and newborn behavior: effect over the first ten days of life. *Pediatrics.* 1976; 58(1):94-100.

Valentine CJ, Hurst NM, Schanler RJ. Hindmilk improves weight gain in low-birth-weight infants fed human milk. *J Pediatr Gastroenterol Nutr.* 1994;18:474-477.

Van Den Bosch CA, Bullough CHW. Effect of early suckling on term neonates' core body temperature. *Ann Trop Paediatr.* 1990;10:347-353.

Vestermark V, Hogdall CK, Birch M, et al. Influence of the mode of delivery on initiation of breastfeeding. *Eur J Obstet Gynecol Repro Biol.* 1991; 38(1):33-38.

Vogel A, Hutchison BF, Mitchell EA. Mastitis in the first year postpartum. *Birth.* 1999;26(4):218-225.

Walker M, Driscoll JW. Sore nipples: the new mother's nemesis. *MCN.* 1989;14:260-265.

Walker M. *Breastfeeding Premature Babies.* Wayne, NJ: Avery Publishing Group; 1990: Lactation Consultant Series, Unit 14.

Walker M. Breastfeeding the sleepy baby. *J Hum Lact.* 1997;13(2):151-153.

Walker, M. Do labor medications affect breastfeeding? *J Hum Lact.* 1997; 12:131-137.

Walker, M. Management of selected early breastfeeding problems seen in clinical practice. *Birth.* 1989;16(3):148-158.

Weatherly-White RCA, et al. Early repair and breastfeeding for infants with cleft lip. *Plast Reconstr Surg.* 1987;79:879-885.

Weber F et al. An ultrasonographic study of the organization of sucking and swallowing by newborn infants. *Dev Med Child Neurol.* 1986;28: 19-24.

Whitelaw A. Kangaroo baby care: just a nice experience or an important advance for preterm infants? *Pediatrics.* 1990;85:604-605.

Wiberg B, Humble K, de Chateau P. Long-term effect on mother-infant behavior of extra contact during the first hour post partum V. Follow-up at three years. *Scand J Soc Med.* 1989;17:181-191.

Widstrom AM, Thingstrom-Paulsson J. The position of the tongue during rooting reflexes elicited in newborn infants before the first suckle. *Acta Paediatr Scand.* 1993;82:281-283.

Widstrom AM, Wahlberg V, et al. Short-term effects of early suckling and touch of the nipple on maternal behavior. *Early Hum Dev.* 1990;21: 153-163.

Wilson NW, Self TW, Hamburger RN. Severe cow's milk induced colitis. *Clin Pediatr.* 1990;29:77-80.

Woodall D, Karas JG. A new light on jaundice: a pilot study. *Clin Pediatr.* 1992;31:353-356.

Woolridge M et al. Individual patterns of milk intake during breastfeeding. *Early Hum Dev.* 1982;4:265-272.

Woolridge M. Aetiology of sore nipples. *Midwifery.* 1986;2:172-176.

Woolridge, M. Anatomy of infant sucking. *Midwifery.* 1986;2:164-171.

Woolridge, M, and Baum, JD. The regulation of human milk flow. In: Lindblad BS. *Perinatal Nutrition.* Vol 6. London: Academic Press; 1988.

Wright AL, Holberg CJ, Martinez FR, Morgan WJ, Taussig LM. Breast-feeding and lower respiratory tract illness in the first year of life. *Br Med J.* 1989;299:946-949.

Yamauchi Y. Hypoglycemia in healthy full-term breastfed neonates during the early days of life: preliminary observation. *Acta Pediatr Japon.* 1997;39(suppl 1):S44-47.

Young J. *Developmental Care of the Premature Baby.* London Balliere Tindall; 1996.

Zeskind PS, Marshall TR, Goff DM. Rhythmic organization of heart rate in breastfed and bottlefed newborn infants. *Early Dev Parenting.* 1992; 1(2):79-87.

Ziemer MM, Cooper DM, Pigeon JG. Evaluation of a dressing to reduce nipple pain and improve nipple skin condition in breastfeeding women. *Nurs Res.* 1995;44(6):347-351.

Ziemer MM, Pigeon JG. Skin changes and pain in the nipple during the first week of lactation. *J Obstet Gynecol Neonatal Nurs.* 1993;22(3): 247-256.

6

Maternal and Infant Pharmacology and Toxicology

In the exam blueprint, 10 to 16 questions are dedicated to maternal and infant pharmacology and toxicology, specifically: maternal use of medications (prescription and OTC drugs, herbs, homeopathic substances); alcohol and tobacco; drugs of abuse; pesticide residues and their effect on the infant, on milk composition, and on lactation.

SUBTOPICS INCLUDED IN THIS CATEGORY

1. Principles of pharmacokinetics
2. Maternal use of medications
    a. Prescription drugs
    b. Herbs and homeopathic substances
    c. Over-the-counter drugs; alcohol, tobacco; dietary drugs
    d. Drugs of abuse
    e. Pesticide residues; environmental toxins
    f. Compounds that affect milk supply
3. Effect on the infant, on milk composition, and on lactation
4. Lactation consultant's role; resources
5. Complementary therapies

CORE READING

Black RF, Jarman L, Simpson J. *Lactation Specialist Self-Study Modules #1-4.* Sudbury, MA: Jones & Bartlett Publishers; 1998: module 4 chap 2A.

Briggs GG, Freeman RK, Yaffe SJ. *Drugs in Pregnancy and Lactation.* 5th ed. Baltimore: Williams & Wilkins; 1998.

Hale T. *Medications and Mothers' Milk.* Amarillo, TX: Pharmasoft Publishing; 1999.

Lauwers J, Shinskie D. *Counseling the Nursing Mother.* 3rd ed, Sudbury, MA: Jones & Bartlett Publishers, 2000: chap 8.

Lawrence RA, Lawrence RM. *Breastfeeding, a Guide for the Medical Profession.* 5th ed. St. Louis: Mosby; 1999: chap 10, appendix D.

Morbacher N, Stock J. *The Breastfeeding Answer Book.* rev ed. Schaumburg, IL: La Leche League International: 1997: chap 24.

Riordan J, Auerbach KG. *Breastfeeding and Human Lactation.* 2nd ed. Sudbury, MA: Jones & Bartlett Publishers; 1999: chap 6.

ADDITIONAL RESOURCES

Albrecht LM, Hatzopoulos FK, eds. Galactopharmacopedia (regular column). *J Hum Lact.* Raleigh NC: International Lactation Consultant Association; 1997.

American Academy of Pediatrics Committee on Drugs. The transfer of drugs and other chemicals into human milk. *Pediatrics.* 1994;93(1):137-150.

Handley R. *Homeopathy for Women.* London: Harper Collins; 1993.

Lawrence RA. A Review of the Medical Benefits and Contraindications to Breastfeeding in the United States (*Maternal and Child Health Technical Information Bulletin*). Arlington, VA: National Center for Education in Maternal and Child Health; October 1997.

McIntyre A. *The Complete Woman's Herbal.* New York, NY: Henry Holt; 1995.

Ullman D, Cummings S. *Everybody's Guide to Homeopathic Medicines,* 1st ed. New York: Jeremy P. Tarcher/Perigree Books; 1991.

Weed S. *Wise Woman Herbal: The Childbearing Year.* New York: Ash Tree Publishing; 1996.

7

Psychology, Sociology, and Anthropology

In the exam blueprint, 10 to 16 questions are dedicated to psychology, sociology, and anthropology, specifically: counseling and adult education skills; grief, postnatal depression, and psychosis; socioeconomic, lifestyle, and employment issues; maternal role adaptation; parenting skills; cultural beliefs and practices; support systems; domestic violence.

SUBTOPICS INCLUDED IN THIS CATEGORY

1. Counseling and adult education skills
2. Grief, postnatal depression, and psychosis
3. Socioeconomic, lifestyle, and employment issues
4. Maternal role adaptation
5. Parenting skills
    a. Cultural beliefs and practices
    b. Support systems
    c. Multiple infants
    d. Sleep issues
6. Domestic violence and abuse

CORE READING

Human Relations Enrichment Workbook. 3rd ed. Schaumburg, IL: La Leche League International; 1994.

Auerbach KG. *Maternal Employment and Breastfeeding.* Wayne, NJ: Avery Publishing Group; 1987: Lactation Consultant Series Unit 6.

Black RF, Jarman L, Simpson J. *Lactation Specialist Self-Study Modules #1-4.* Sudbury, MA: Jones & Bartlett Publishers, 1998: module 1 chap 1A, B, & C; chap 3B; module 4 chap 1A, 3B.

Bocar DL, Moore K. *Acquiring the Parental Role: a Theoretical Perspective.* Wayne, NJ: Avery Publishing Group; 1987: Lactation Consultant Series, Unit 16.

Gromada KK. *Mothering Multiples: Breastfeeding and Care for Twins or More!* 2nd ed. Schaumburg IL: La Leche League International; 1999.

Herforth D. *Counseling Grieving Families.* Wayne, NJ: Avery Publishing Group; 1986; Lactation Consultant Series, Unit 12.

Klaus MH, Kennell JH, Klaus PH. *Bonding: Building the Foundations of Secure Attachment and Independence.* St. Louis: Mosby; 1995.

Lauwers J, Shinskie D. *Counseling the Nursing Mother.* 3rd ed. Sudbury, MA: Jones & Bartlett Publishers, 2000: chaps 1, 3, 4, 9, 17, 18, 21, 22, 23.

Lawrence RA. *Breastfeeding, a Guide for the Medical Profession.* 5th ed. St. Louis: Mosby; 1994: chaps 10, 13, 21, appendix K.

Morbacher N, Stock J. *The Breastfeeding Answer Book.* rev ed. Schaumburg, IL: La Leche League International: 1997: chaps 1, 15.

Riordan J, Auerbach KG. *Breastfeeding and Human Lactation.* 2nd ed. Sudbury, MA: Jones & Bartlett Publishers; 1999: chaps 1, 2, 3, 10, 18.

Savage F. *Helping Mothers to Breastfeed.* Nairobi, Kenya: African Medical and Research Foundation; 1994.

Small MF. *Our Babies, Ourselves: How Biology and Culture Shape the Way We Parent.* New York: Random House; 1998.

Stuart-Macadam P, Dettwyler KA. *Breastfeeding: Biocultural Perspectives.* New York: Aldine De Gruyter; 1995: chaps 3, 4, 5, 7, 10, 13, 14.

Taylor MM. *Transcultural Aspects of Breastfeeding—USA.* Wayne, NJ: Avery Publishing Group; 1985: Lacation Consultant Series, Unit 2.

ADDITIONAL RESOURCES

_____. *Best Start's Three Step Counseling Strategy.* Tampa, FL: Best Start Social Marketing, 1997.

Arlotti JP, Cottrell BH, Lee SH, Curtin JJ. Breastfeeding among low-income women with and without peer support. *J Community Health Nurs.* 1998;15(3):163-178.

Auerbach KG, Guss E. Maternal employment and breastfeeding: A study of 567 women's experiences. *Am J Dis Child.* 1984;138:958-960.

Auerbach KG. Employed breastfeeding mothers: problems they encounter. *Birth.* 1984;11(1):17-20.

Auerbach KG. Scheduled feedings ... is this "God's Order?" *J Perinat Ed.* 1998;7(3):1-6.

Baumgarner NJ. *Mothering Your Nursing Toddler.* Revised Ed. Shaumburg, IL: LaLeche League International; 2000.

Baumslag N, Michels D. *Milk, Money, and Madness:* Westport CT: Bergin & Garvey; 1995: chaps 1, 6.

Beck CT. A checklist to identify women at risk for developing postpartum depression. *JOGNN.* 1998;27:39-46.

Beck CT. Postpartum onset of panic disorder. *Image: J Nurs Scholarship.* 1998;30:131-135.

Beck CT. The effects of postpartum depression on maternal-infant interaction: A meta-analysis. *Nurs Re.* 1995;44:298-304.

Beck CT. The lived experience of postpartum depression: a phenomenological study. *Nurs Res.* 1992;41:166-170.

Belenky MF, Clinchy BM, Goldberger NR, Tarule JM. *Women's Ways of Knowing.* New York: Basic Books; 1986.

Bertelsen C, Auerbach KG. *Nutrition and Breastfeeding: The Cultural Connection.* Wayne, NJ: Avery Publishing Group; 1987: Lactation Consultant Series Unit 11.

Bing E, Colman L. *Laughter and Tears: the Emotional Life of New Mothers.* New York: Henry Holt; 1997.

Blum, Barbara L. *Psychological Aspects of Pregnancy, Birth and Bonding.* New York: Human Sciences Press; 1980.

Borg S, Lasker J. *When Pregnancy Fails.* Boston: Beacon Press; 1981.

Bridges CB, Frank DI, Curtin J. Employer attitudes toward breastfeeding in the workplace. *J Hum Lact.* 1997;13(3):215-219.

Buckley KM. Beliefs and practices related to extended breastfeeding among La Leche League mothers. *J Perina Ed.* 1992;1(2):45-53.

Buckner E, Matsubara M. Support network utilization by breastfeeding mothers: *J Hum Lact.* 1993;9(4):231-235.

Cohen R, Mrtek MB, Mrtek RG. Comparison of maternal absenteeism and infant illness rates among breastfeeding women and formula-feeding women in two corporations. *Am J Health Prom.* 1995;10(2):148-153.

Cohen R, Mrtek MB. The impact of two corporate lactation programs on incidence and duration by breastfeeding mothers. *Am J Health.* 1994; 8(6):436-441.

Coreil J, Bryant CA, Westover BJ, Bailey D. Health professionals and breastfeeding counseling: client and provider views. *J Hum Lact.* 1995; 11(4):265-271.

Da Vanzo J, Starbird E, Leibowitz A. Do women's breastfeeding experiences with their first-borns affect whether they breastfeed their subsequent children? *Soc Biol.* 1990;37(3-4):223-232.

Dodgson JE, Duckett L. Breastfeeding in the workplace. Building a support program for nursing mothers. *AAOHN J.* 1997;45(6):290-298.

Eidelman, Al, Hoffman, NW, Kaitz M: Cognitive deficits in women after childbirth. *Obstet Gynecol.* 1993;81:764-776.

Freed GL, Clark SJ, Harris BG, Lowdermilk DL. Methods and outcomes of breastfeeding instruction for nursing students. *J Hum Lact.* 1996;12(2): 105-110.

Freed GL, et al. Attitudes and education of pediatric house staff concerning breast-feeding. *South Med J.* 1992;85(5):483-485.

Freed GL, et al. Breast-feeding education and practice in family medicine. *J Fam Pract.* 1995;40(3):263-269.

Freed GL, et al. National assessment of physicians' breast-feeding knowledge, attitudes, training, and experience. *JAMA.* 1995;273(6):472-476.

Freed GL, et al. Breast-feeding education of obstetrics-gynecology residents and practitioners. *Am J Obstet Gynecol.* 1995;173(5):1607-1613.

Freed GL, et al. Pediatrician involvement in breast-feeding promotion: a national study of residents and practitioners. *Pediatrics.* 1995;96(3 Pt 1): 490-494.

Goldstein AO, et al. Breast-feeding counseling practices of family practice residents. *Fam Med.* 1993;25(8):524-529.

Gromada KK, Spangler AK. Breastfeeding twins and higher-order multiples. *JOGNN.* 1998;27:441-449.

Gromada KK. Breastfeeding more than one: multiples and tandem breastfeeding. *NAACOG's (AWHONN's) Clin Issues Perina Women's Health Nurs.* 1992;3:656-666.

Gromada KK. Maternal-infants attachment: the first step toward individualizing twins. *MCN.* 1981;6:129-134.

Haider R, Begum S. Working women, maternity entitlements, and breastfeeding: a report from Bangladesh. *J Hum Lact.* 1995;11(4):273-277.

Hauck Y, Reinbold J. Criteria for successful breastfeeding: mothers' perceptions. *J Aust Coll Midwives.* 1996;9(1):21-27.

Hewat RJ, Ellis DJ. Breastfeeding as a maternal-child team effort: women's self-perceptions. *Health Care Woman Int.* 1984;5:437-452.

Hordern BB. Breastfeeding and the bottom line. *Working Woman.* 1994; 19(4):18.

Ilse S. *Empty Arms: Coping with Miscarriage. Stillbirth, and Infant Death.* Maple Plain, MN: Wintergreen Press 1992.

Jakobsen MS, Sodemann M, Molbak K, Aaby P. Reason for termination of breastfeeding and the length of breastfeeding. *Int J Epidemio.* 1996; 25(1):115-121.

Jones EG, Matheney RJ. Relationship between infant feeding and exclusion from child care because of illness. *J Am Diet Assoc.* 1993;93(7):809-811.

Kendall-Tackett KA, Sugarman M. The social consequences of long-term breastfeeding. *J Hum Lact.* 1995;11(3):179-183.

Kennell J, Klaus M, McGrath S, Robertson S, Hinkley C. Continuous emotional support during labor in a U.S. hospital. A randomized controlled trial. *JAMA.* 1991;265(17):2197-2201.

Kennell JH, et al. Bonding: recent observations that alter perinatal care. *Pediatr Rev.* 1998;19(1):4-12.

Kennell H. The time has come to reassess delivery room routines. *Birth.* 1994;21:1:49-51.

Kitzinger S. *Women as Mothers: How They See Themselves in Different Cultures.* New York: Vintage Books; 1978.

Klaus M. Mother and infant: early emotional ties. *Pediatrics.* 1998;102(5): 1244-1246.

Kurinki N, Shiono PH, Ezrine SF, Rhoads GG. Does maternal employment affect breastfeeding? *Am J Pub Health.* 1989;79:1247-1250.

Locklin MP, Naber, SJ. Does breastfeeding empower women? Insights from a select group of educated, low-income, minority women. *Birth.* 1993; 20(1):30-35.

Matthews K, Webber K, McKim E, Banoub-Baddour S, Laryea M. Maternal infant-feeding decisions: reasons and influences. *Can J Nurs Res.* 1998;30(2):177-198.

McKenna JJ, Thoman EB, Anders TF, Sadeh A, Schectman VL & Glotzbach SF. Pediatric Review: Infant-parent co-sleeping in an evolutionary perspective: implications for understanding infant sleep development and the sudden infant death syndrome. *Sleep.* 1993;16(3):263-282.

Mercer RT, et al. Maternal-infant attachment of experienced and inexperienced mothers during infancy. *Nurs Res.* 1994;43(6):344-351.

Mercer RT. Factors impacting on the maternal role the first year of motherhood. *Birth Defects Orig Artic Ser.* 1981;17(6):233-252.

Miller, Alice. *For Your Own Good: Hidden Cruelty In Child-Rearing And The Roots Of Violence.* New York: Farrar, Straus, Giroux; 1984.

Morse JM, Harrison MJ. Social coercion for weaning. *J Nurs Midwife.* 1987;32:205-210.

Moscone SR, Moore MJ. Breastfeeding during pregnancy. *J Hum Lact.* 1993;9(2):83-88.

Mulford C. Swimming upstream: breastfeeding care in a nonbreastfeeding culture. *JOGNN.* 1995;24(5):464-474.

Mundal LD. et al. Maternal-infant separation at birth among substance using pregnant women: implications for attachment. *Soc Work Health Care.* 1991;16(1):133-143.

Newton N. *Maternal Emotions.* New York: Paul E. Hoeber, 1955.

Newton N. Trebly sensuous woman. *Psych Today.* 1971;5:68-71, 98-99.

Palmer G. *The Politics of Breastfeeding.* 2nd ed. London: Pandora Press; 1993.

Panuthos C, Romeo C. *Ended Beginnings: Healing Childbearing Losses.* South Hadley, MA; Bergin & Garvey Publishers; 1984.

Peterson G, Mehl L. Some determinants of mother attachments. *Am J Psychiatry.* 1978;135:1168-1173.

Poore M, Foster JC. Epidural and no epidural anesthesia: differences between mothers and their experience of birth. *Birth.* 1985;12(4):205-219.

Pridham KF, Chang AS. Transition to being a mother of a new infant in the first 3 months: maternal problem solving and self-appraisals. *J Adv Nurs.* 1992;17:204-216.

Reamer SB, Sugarman M. Breastfeeding beyond six months: mothers' perception of the positive and negative consequences. *J Trop Pediatr.* 1987; 33:93-97.

Riordan JM, Rapp ET. Pleasure and purpose—the sensuousness of breastfeeding. *JOGN Nurs.* 1980;9:109-112.

Rodriguez-Garcia R, Frazier L. Cultural paradoxes relating to sexuality and breastfeeding. *J Human Lact.* 1995;11(2):111-115.

Rubin R. *Maternal Identity and the Maternal Experience.* New York: Spring Publishing; 1984.

Saint L, Maggiore P, Hartmann PE. Yield and nutrient content of milk in eight women breast-feeding twins and triplets. *B J Nutr.* 1986;56:49-58.

Samuel J. Breastfeeding and the empowerment of women. *Can Nurse.* 1997;93(2):47-48.

Satir V. *The New Peoplemaking.* Mountain View, CA: Science and Behavior Books, Inc., 1988.

Schafer E, Vogel MK, Viegas S, Hausafus C. Volunteer peer counselors increase breastfeeding duration among rural low-income women. *Birth.* 1998;25(2):101-106.

Sikorski J, Renfrew MJ. Support for breastfeeding mothers (Cochran Review). In: *The Cochrane Library.* Issue 1. Oxford: Update Software; 1999.

Sosa R, et al. The effect of a supportive companion on perinatal problems, length of labor, and mother-infant interaction. *N Engl J Med.* 1980; 303(11):597-600.

Taylor MM. *Transcultural Aspects of Breastfeeding—USA.* Wayne, NJ; Avery Publishing Group; 1985: Lactation Consultant Series, Unit 2.

Van Esterik P, Menon L. *Being Mother-Friendly: A Practical Guide For Working Women And Breastfeeding.* Penang, Malaysia: World Alliance For Breastfeeding Action; 1996.

Van Esterik P. *Women, Work, and Breastfeeding.* North York, Ontario: York University Press; 1994.

Veronnen P: Breastfeeding- reasons for giving up and transient lactational crises. *Acta Paediatr Scand.* 1982;71:447-450.

Virden SF. The relationship between infant feeding method and maternal role adjustment. *J Nurs Midwife.* 1988;33:31-35.

Widstrom AM, Wahlberg V, et al. Short-term effects of early suckling and touch of the nipple on maternal behavior. *Early Hum Dev.* 1990;21: 153-163.

Wilton JM. Breastfeeding Multiples. In Keith LG, Papiernik E, Keith DM, Luke B, eds. *Multiple Pregnancy: Epidemiology, Gestation, And Perinatal Outcome.* New York: Parthenon; 1995.

Winnicott DW. *Babies And Their Mothers,* Reading, MA: Addison-Wesley; 1987.

Wismont JM, et al. The lesbian childbearing experience: assessing developmental tasks. *Image J Nurs Sch.* 1989;21(3):137-141.

Wrigley EA, Hutchinson SA. Long-term breastfeeding: the secret bond. *J Nurs Midwife.* 1990;35:35-41.

8

Growth Parameters and Developmental Milestones

In the exam blueprint, 10 to 16 questions are dedicated to growth parameters and developmental milestones, specifically: growth patterns, recognition of normal/delayed physical, psychological, and cognitive developmental milestones.

SUBTOPICS INCLUDED IN THIS CATEGORY

1. Growth patterns; growth curves
2. Recognition of normal and delayed developmental milestones
   a. Physical, including failure to thrive and slow to gain
   b. Psychological
   c. Cognitive
3. Common breastfeeding behaviors and patterns (normal)
   a. Sleep patterns
   b. Weaning
   c. Breastfeeding during pregnancy; tandem nursing

CORE READING

Black RF, Jarman L, Simpson J. *Lactation Specialist Self-Study Modules #1-4.* Sudbury, MA: Jones & Bartlett Publishers; 1998: module 4 chap 1B.

Cunningham AS, Jelliffe DB, Jelliffe EFP. *Breastfeeding, Growth and Illness: an Annotated Bibliography.* New York: UNICEF; 1992.

Lauwers J, Shinskie D. *Counseling the Nursing Mother.* 3rd ed. Sudbury, MA: Jones & Bartlett Publishers; 2000: chap 16.

Lawrence RA. *Breastfeeding, a Guide for the Medical Profession,* 5th ed. St. Louis: Mosby; 1994: chap 12, appendix J.

Morbacher N, Stock J. *The Breastfeeding Answer Book.* rev ed. Schaumburg, IL: La Leche League International; 1997: chap 6.

Riordan J, Auerbach KG. *Breastfeeding and Human Lactation,* 2nd ed. Sudbury, MA: Jones & Bartlett Publishers; 1999: chaps 11, 19.

Sears W, Sears M. *The Baby Book: Everything You Need to Know About Your Baby From Birth to Age Two.* Boston: Little, Brown; 1993.

Stuart-Macadam P, Dettwyler KA. *Breastfeeding: Biocultural Perspectives.* New York: Aldine De Gruyter; 1995: chaps 3, 4, 5, 7, 10, 13, 14.

Whaley LF, Wong DL. *Nursing Care of Infants and Children,* 4th ed. St. Louis: Mosby; 1991: unit II.

ADDITIONAL RESOURCES

_____. *An Evaluation of Infant Growth.* Geneva: World Health Organization Nutrition Unit; 1994.

_____. *The Womanly Art of Breastfeeding.* 6th rev ed. Schaumburg, IL: La Leche League International; 1997.

Als H. *Manual for the Naturalistic Observation of Newborn Behavior* (Preterm and Fullterm Infants). Boston: The Children's Hospital; 1981; 1984 revision.

Butte NF, Wills C, Jean CA, Smith EO, Garza C. Feeding patterns of exclusively breastfed infants during the first four months of life. *Early Hum Dev.* 1985;12(3):291-300.

Dewey KG, Heinig J, Nommsen-Rivers L. Differences in morbidity between breastfed and formula-fed infants. *J Pediatr.* 1995;126:696-702.

Dewey KG, Heinig MJ, Nommsen LA, Lonnerdal B. Maternal versus infant factors related to breastmilk intake and residual milk volume: the DARLING study. *Pediatrics.* 1991;87(6):829-837.

Dewey KG, Heinig MJ, Nommsen LA, Peerson JM, Lonnerdal B. Breastfed infants are leaner than formula-fed infants at 1y of age: the DARLING study. *Am J Clin Nutr.* 1993;57:140-145.

Dewey KG, Heinig MJ, Nommsen LA, Peerson JM, Lonnerdal B. Growth of breastfed and formula-fed infants from 0 to 18 months: the DARLING study. *Pediatrics.* 1992;89:1035-1041.

Diaz S, Herreros C, Aravena R, et al. Breastfeeding duration and growth of fully breastfed infants in a poor urban Chilean population. *Am J Clin Nutr.* 1995;62(2):371-376.

Dubignon J, Cooper D. Good and poor feeding behavior in the neonatal period. *Infant Behav Dev.* 1980;3:395-408.

Elias MF, Nicolson NA, Bora C, Johnston J. Sleep/wake patterns of breastfed infants in the first 2 years of life. *Pediatrics.* 1986;77:322-329.

Fildes V. *Breasts, Bottles and Babies: a History of Infant Feeding.* Edinburgh: Edinburgh University Press; 1986.

Fildes V. *Wet Nursing: a history from antiquity to the present.* New York: Basil Blackwell; 1988.

Foman SJ. *Nutrition of Normal Infants.* St. Louis: Mosby; 1993.

Gulick E. The effects of breastfeeding on toddler health. *Pediatr Nurs.* Jan-Feb 1986.

Heinig MH, Nommsen LA, Peerson MH, Lonnerdal B, Dewey KG. Energy and protein intakes of breastfed and formula-fed infants during the first year of life and their association with growth velocity: the DARLING study. *Am J Clin Nutr.* 1993;58:152-161.

Hendricks KM. Weaning recommendations: the scientific basis. *Nutr Rev.* 1992;50(5):125-133.

Hervada AR, Newman Dr. Weaning: historical perspectives, practical recommendations, and current controversies. *Current Prob Pediatr.* 1992; 22(5):223-241.

Huggins K, Ziedrich L. *The Nursing Mother's Guide to Weaning.* Boston: The Harvard Common Press; 1994.

Institute of Medicine (Subcommittee on Nutrition during Lactation, Food and Nutrition Board). *Nutrition during Lactation.* Washington DC: National Academy of Sciences; 1991.

Kleinman RE, ed. *Pediatric Nutrition Handbook.* 4th ed. Elk Grove Village IL: American Academy of Pediatrics; 1998.

Osofsky, Joy Doniger. *Handbook of Infant Development.* New York: John Wiley & Sons; 1987.

Paul K, Dittrichova J, Papousek H. Infant feeding behavior: development in patterns and motivation. *Dev. Psycholbiol.* Nov 1996;29(7):563-576.

Pryor K, Pryor G. *Nursing Your Baby.* New York: Pocket Books; 1991: chaps 1, 5, 6, 10, 11, 12, 14.

Quillin Sl. Infant and mother sleep patterns during 4th postpartum week. *Issues Compr Pediatr Nurs.* Apr 1997;20(2):115-123.

Whitehead RG. The human weaning process. *Pediatrics.* 1985; 75(suppl): 189-193.

Wright P, MacLeod HA, Cooper MJ. Waking at night: the effect of early feeding experience. *Child Care Health Dev.* Nov 1983;9(6):309-319.

Wright P. Learning experiences in feeding behaviour during infancy. *J Psychosom Res.* 1988;32(6):613-619.

Yamauchi Y, Yamanouchi I. Breastfeeding frequency during the first 24 hours after birth in full-term neonates. August 1990; *Pediatrics.* 86(2): 171-175.

Interpretation of Research

In the exam blueprint, 4 to 8 questions are dedicated to interpretation of research, specifically: skills required for critical appraisal of research literature; LC educational materials and consumer literature; knowledge of terminology used in research and basic statistics; and surveys and data collection for research purposes.

SUBTOPICS INCLUDED IN THIS CATEGORY

1. Skills required for critical appraisal of research literature
   a. Terminology
   b. Design, human rights
   c. Measurement tools
2. Knowledge of terminology used in research and basic statistics
3. Surveys and data collection for research purposes
4. LC educational materials and consumer literature

CORE READING

Fredrickson D. Breastfeeding study design problems—health policy, epidemiologic and pediatric perspectives. In: Stuart-Macadam P, Dettwyler KA. *Breastfeeding: Biocultural Perspectives.* New York: Aldine De Gruyter; 1995.

Lauwers J, Shinskie D. *Counseling the Nursing Mother,* 3rd ed. Sudbury, MA: Jones & Bartlett Publishers, 2000: chaps 9, 10, 25.

Lawrence RA, Lawrence RM. *Breastfeeding, a Guide for the Medical Profession.* 5th ed. St. Louis: Mosby; 1999: chapter 22, appendix M.

Morbacher N, Stock J. *The Breastfeeding Answer Book.* rev ed. Schaumburg, IL: La Leche League International; 1997: chap 24.

Riordan J, Auerbach KG. *Breastfeeding and Human Lactation.* 2nd ed. Sudbury, MA: Jones & Bartlett Publishers; 1999: chaps 8, 23, appendices I, K, L.

ADDITIONAL RESOURCES

Armstrong HC. International recommendations for consistent breastfeeding definitions. *J Hum Lact.* 1991;7:51-54.

Auerbach KG. Beyond the issue of accuracy: evaluating patient education materials for breastfeeding mothers. *J Hum Lact.* 1988;4:108-110.

Bennett KJ, et al. A controlled trial of teaching critical appraisal of the clinical literature to medical students. *JAMA.* 1987;257(11):1275.

Burns N, Grove SK. *The Practice of Nursing Research: Conduct, Critique and Utilization,* 3rd ed. Philadelphia: Saunders; 1997.

Downs FS. *Handbook of Research Methodology.* New York: American Journal of Nursing Company; 1988.

Evidence-Based Medicine Working Group. Evidence-based medicine: a new approach to teaching the practice of medicine. *JAMA.* 1992;268(17):2420.

Frank-Stromberg M, Olsen SJ. *Instruments for Clinical Health-Care Research,* 2nd ed. Sudbury, MA: Jones & Bartlett Publishers; 1997.

Fredrickson D. Breastfeeding study design problems—health policy, epidemiologic and pediatric perspectives. In: Stuart-Macadam P, Dettwyler KA. *Breastfeeding: Biocultural Perspectives.* New York: Aldine De Gruyter; 1995.

Goer H. *Obstetric Myths versus Research Realities: A Guide To The Medical Literature.* Westport CT: Bergin & Garvey; 1995.

Gravetter FJ, Wallnau LB. *Statistics for the Behavioral Sciences,* 3rd ed. St. Paul, MN: West Publishing; 1992.

Greenhalgh T. How to read a paper: assessing the methodological quality of published papers. *Br Med J.* 1997a;315:305.

Greenhalgh T. How to read a paper: getting your bearing (deciding what the paper is about). *Br Med J.* 1997b;315:243.

Greenhalgh T. How to read a paper: papers that go beyond numbers (qualitative research). *Br Med J.* 1997c;315:740.

Greenhalgh T. How to read a paper: papers that summarize other papers (systematic reviews and meta-analyses). *Br Med J.* 1997d;315:672.

Greenhalgh T. How to read a paper: statistics for the non-statistician II: significant relationships and their pitfalls. *Br Med J.* 1997e;315:422.

Greenhalgh T. How to read a paper: the Medline database. *Br Med J.* 1997f;315:180.

Grimes DA. How can we translate good science into good perinatal care? *Birth.* 1986;13(2):83-90.

Grimes DA. Introducing evidence-based medicine into a department of obstetrics and gynecology. *Obstet Gynecol.* 1995;86(3):451.

Labbok M, Krasovek K. Toward consistency in breastfeeding definitions. *Stud Fam Plann.* 1990;21:226-230.

Malec MA. *Essential Statistics for Social Research.* Philadelphia: J.B. Lippincott; 1977.

Polit DF, Hungler BP. *Nursing Research Principles and Methods.* 5th ed. Philadelphia: J.B. Lippincott; 1995.

Riordan J. Readable, relevant, and reliable: the three Rs of breastfeeding pamphlets. *Breastfeed Abst.* 1985;5:5-6.

Smith L. A scoresheet for evaluating breastfeeding educational materials. *J Hum Lact.* 1995;11(4):307-311.

10

Ethical and Legal Issues

In the exam blueprint, 4 to 8 questions are dedicated to ethical and legal issues, specifically: IBLCE Code of Ethics; standards of practice; medical and legal responsibilities; report writing skills; record keeping; referrals and interdisciplinary relationships; neglect and maternal/infant abuse.

SUBTOPICS INCLUDED IN THIS CATEGORY

1. IBLCE Code of Ethics
2. Standards of practice
3. Medical and legal responsibilities; informed consent
4. Report writing skills; record keeping
5. Referrals and interdisciplinary relationships
   a. Complementary and alternative therapies
   b. Neglect and maternal/infant abuse

CORE READING

_____. *Code of Ethics.* Falls Church VA: International Board of Lactation Consultant Examiners; 1996.

_____. *Position Paper on Infant Feeding.* Raleigh NC: International Lactation Consultant Association; 1994.

_____. *Standards of Practice for Lactation Consultants.* Raleigh NC: International Lactation Consultant Association; 1995.

Baumslag N, Michels D. *Milk, Money and Madness.* Westport CT: Bergin & Garvey; 1995.

Bornmann PG. *Legal Considerations and the Lactation Consultant—U.S.A.* Wayne, NJ: Avery Publishing Group; 1986: Lactation Consultant Series, Unit 3.

Lauwers J, Shinskie D. *Counseling the Nursing Mother.* 3rd ed. Sudbury, MA: Jones & Bartlett Publishers; 2000: chaps 2, 10, 24.

Lawrence RA. *Breastfeeding, a Guide for the Medical Profession.* 5th ed. St. Louis: Mosby; 1999: chap 1, appendix M.

Palmer G. *The Politics of Breastfeeding.* 2nd ed. London: Pandora Press; 1993.

Riordan J, Auerbach KG. *Breastfeeding and Human Lactation,* 2nd ed. Sudbury, MA: Jones & Bartlett Publishers; 1999: chap 22, appendices D, G, H, J.

Stuart-Macadam P, Dettwyler KA. *Breastfeeding: Biocultural Perspectives.* New York: Aldine De Gruyter; 1995: chap 6.

ADDITIONAL RESOURCES

_____. *Protecting, Promoting and Supporting Breastfeeding: The Special Role of Maternity Services.* A Joint WHO/UNICEF statement. Geneva: World Health Organization Nutrition Unit; 1989.

_____. *Standards of Practice for Lactation Consultants.* Raleigh NC: International Lactation Consultant Association; 1999.

American Academy of Pediatrics Work Group on Breastfeeding, 1997. Breastfeeding and the use of Human Milk. *Pediatrics.* 1997;100:1035-1039. (Policy # RE9729)

American College of Nurse-Midwives. Promoting breastfeeding among vulnerable mothers. *Nurse-Midwifery.* 1993;38(1):1-4.

American Hospital Association Section for Maternal and Child Health: *Promotion of Breastfeeding.* Chicago: Am Hosp Assn Dec 1992.

Amery J, Tomkins A. Advertising infant formulas in hospitals. *BMJ* Nov 23 1991;303(6813):1336.

Annual Report from the Advisory Panel on the Marketing in Australia of Infant Formula, July 1996-June 1997. Commonwealth of Australia, 1997.

ASPO/Lamaze Position Paper on Infant Feeding. Washington DC: Lamaze International (formerly ASPO/Lamaze); 1991.

AWHONN Committee on Practice. Guideline for Breastfeeding Support. In *Guidelines and Standards.* Washington DC: Association of Women's Health, Obstetric, and Neonatal Nursing; 1998.

Bergevin Y, Dougherty C, Kramer MS. Do infant formula samples shorten the duration of breastfeeding? *Lancet.* 1983;1(8334):1148-1151.

Blake RL Jr, et al. Patients' attitudes about gifts to physicians from pharmaceutical companies. *J Am Board Fam Pract.* 1995;8(6):457-464.

Bliss MC, Wilkie J, Acredolo C, Berman S, Tebb KP. The effect of discharge pack formula and breast pumps on breastfeeding duration and choice of infant feeding method. *Birth.* 1997;24(2):90-97.

Breastfeeding: The Technical Basis And Recommendations For Action. Geneva: World Health Organization; 1993.

Cadwell K. *Growing the Breastfeeding Friendly Community.* Weston MA: National Alliance for Breastfeeding Advocacy; 1996.

Centers for Disease Control and Prevention, 1994. Guidelines for preventing transmission of human immunodeficiency virus through transplantation of human tissue and organs. *MMWR.* May 20, 1994;43(RR-8): 1-7.

Chalmers I. Minimizing harm and maximizing benefit during innovation in health care: controlled or uncontrolled experiment? *Birth.* 1986;13(3): 155-164.

Chren MM, Landefeld CS, Murray TH. Doctors, drug companies, and gifts. *JAMA.* 1989;262:3448-3451.

Edwards MA. The Lactation Consultant: A New Profession. *Birth.* 1985; 12(3)suppl:9-11.

Emanuel EJ, Emanuel LL. Four models of the physician-patient relationship. *JAMA.* 1992;267(16):2221-2226.

Frank DA, et al. Commercial discharge packs and breastfeeding counseling: Effects of infant feeding practices in a randomized trial. *Pediatrics.* 1987; 80:845-854.

Freed GL, et al. Attitudes and education of pediatric house staff concerning breast-feeding. *South Med J.* 1992;85(5):483-485.

Freed GL, et al. Breast-feeding education and practice in family medicine. *J Fam Pract.* 1995;40(3):263-269.

Freed GL, et al. National assessment of physicians' breast-feeding knowledge, attitudes, training, and experience. *JAMA.* 1995;273(6):472-476.

Freed GL, et al. Breast-feeding education of obstetrics-gynecology residents and practitioners. *Am J Obstet Gynecol.* 1995;173(5):1607-1613.

Freed GL, et al. Pediatrician involvement in breast-feeding promotion: a national study of residents and practitioners. *Pediatrics.* 1995;96(3 Pt 1): 490-494.

Freed GL. Breastfeeding: time to teach what we preach. *JAMA.* 1993;269: 243-245.

Gartner LM, Newton ER. Breastfeeding: role of the obstetrician. *ACOG Clin Rev.* 1998;3(1).

Gosha J, Brucker MC. A Self-Help Group for New Mothers: An Evaluation. *Matern Child Nurs.* 1986;11:20-23.

Greer FR, Apple RD. Physicians, formula companies and advertising. *Am J Dis Child.* 1991;145:282-286.

Hartlaub PP, Wolkenstein AS, Laufenburg HF. Obtaining informed consent: it is not simply asking "do you understand?" *J Fam Pract.* 1993; 36(4):383-384.

Hauth JC, Merenstein GB, Eds. *Guidelines for Perinatal Care.* 4th ed. Elk Grove Village, IL: American Academy of Pediatrics; Washington DC: American College of Obstetricians and Gynecologists; 1997.

Heinig J. Closet consulting and other enabling behaviors. *J Hum Lact.* 1998;14(4): Editor's Note.

Howard CR, et al. Infant formula distribution and advertising in pregnancy: a hospital survey. *Birth.* 1994;21(1):14-19.

Howard CR, Schaffer SJ, Lawrence RA. Attitudes, practices, and recommendations by obstetricians about infant feeding. *Birth.* 1997;24(4): 240-246.

Howard FM, Howard CR, Weitzman M. The physician as advertiser: the unintentional discouragement of breast-feeding. *Obstet Gynecol.* 1993; 81(6):1048-1051.

ICEA Position Paper on Infant Feeding. Minneapolis MN: International Childbirth Education Association; 1992.

ILCA *Position Paper on Infant Feeding.* Raleigh NC: International Lactation Consultant Association; 1994.

Innocenti Declaration on the Protection, Promotion, and Support of Breastfeeding. Florence, Italy: 1990.

International Code of Marketing of Breast-Milk Substitutes. Geneva: World Health Organization; 1981.

Kleinman RE, ed. *Pediatric Nutrition Handbook.* 4th ed. Elk Grove Village, IL: American Academy of Pediatrics; 1998.

Margolis LH. The ethics of accepting gifts from pharmaceutical companies. *Pediatrics.* 1991;88(6):1233-1237.

McIntyre E. Breastfeeding management: helping the mother help herself. *Breastfeed Rev.* 1991:129-132.

Miller NH, Miller DJ, Chism M. Breastfeeding practices among resident physicians. *Pediatrics.* 1996;98:434-437.

National Center for Infectious Diseases, Centers for Disease Control and Prevention. Perspectives in Disease Prevention and Health Promotion Update: Universal Precautions for Prevention of Transmission of Human Immunodeficiency Virus, Hepatitis B Virus, and Other Bloodborne Pathogens in Health-Care Settings. *MMWR.* June 24, 1988;37(24): 377-388.

National Center for Infectious Diseases, Centers for Disease Control and Prevention. Public Health Service Guidelines for the Management of Health-Care Worker Exposures to HIV and Recommendations for Postexposure Prophylaxis. *MMWR.* May 15, 1998;47(RR-7):1-28.

NAPNAP Position Statement on Breastfeeding. *J Pediatr Health Care.* 1993;7:289.

National Association of WIC Directors (NAWD) Guidelines for Breastfeeding Promotion and Support in the WIC program. Washington DC: NAWD; 1994.

Nursing Practice Resource on Facilitating Breastfeeding. Nurses Association of the American College of Obstetricians and Gynecologists (NAACOG). Nov 1991.

Position of the American Dietetic Association: Promotion of breastfeeding. *JADA.* 1997;97:662-666.

Promotion of breastfeeding: Recommendations of the Councils of the Society for Pediatric Research (SPR) and American Pediatric Society (APS), and of the American Academy of Pediatrics (AAP). *Pediatr Res.* 1982;16: 264-265.

Recommendations of The International Federation of Gynecology and Obstetrics for Actions to Encourage Breastfeeding. *Int J Gynecol Obstet.* 1982;20:171-172.

Snell BJ, Krantz M, Keeton R, Delgado K, Peckham C. The association of formula samples given at hospital discharge with the early duration of breastfeeding. *J Hum Lact.* 1992;8(2):67-72. Published erratum appears in *J Hum Lact.* 1992;8(3):135.

Statement of policy [on breastfeeding]. International Confederation of Midwives, Chiswick, London, Engalnd.

Sullivan P. CMA supports breastfeeding, "condemns" contracts between formula makers, hospitals. *Can Med Assoc J.* 1992;146(9):1610-1612.

Van Esterik, P. *Beyond the Breast-Bottle Controversy.* New Brunswick NJ: Rutgers University Press; 1989.

Waggett GG, Waggett RR. Breast is best: legislation supporting is an absolute bare necessity—a model approach. *Maryland J Contemp Legal Issues.* 1995;6(1).

Young EWD. *Alpha and Omega: Ethics at the Frontier of Life and Death.* Reading, MA: Addison-Wesley; 1989.

11

Breastfeeding Equipment and Technology

In the exam blueprint, 10 to 16 questions are dedicated to breastfeeding equipment and technology, specifically: breastfeeding equipment and technology; identification of breastfeeding devices and equipment, appropriate use, and technical expertise in using them properly; milk banking.

SUBTOPICS INCLUDED IN THIS CATEGORY

1. Identification of breastfeeding devices and equipment
   a. Milk expression/removal devices
   b. Feeding devices
   c. Other devices, including social
   d. Other remedies and therapies
2. Appropriate use and technical expertise in using them properly
3. Donor human milk banking

CORE READING

Black RF, Jarman L, Simpson J. *Lactation Specialist Self-Study Modules #1-4.* Sudbury, MA: Jones & Bartlett Publishers; 1998: module 2, chap 3B.

Frantz, K. *Breastfeeding Product Guide.* Sundland, CA: Geddes Productions; 1994.

Lauwers J, Shinskie D. *Counseling the Nursing Mother,* 3rd ed. Sudbury, MA: Jones & Bartlett Publishers; 2000: chaps 5, 19.

Lawrence RA, Lawrence RM. *Breastfeeding, a Guide for the Medical Profession.* 5th ed. St. Louis: Mosby; 1999: chap 20, appendix F.

Morbacher N, Stock J. *The Breastfeeding Answer Book.* rev. ed. Schaumburg, IL: La Leche League International; 1997: appendix: breast pumps.

Riordan J, Auerbach KG. *Breastfeeding and Human Lactation,* 2nd ed. Sudbury, MA: Jones & Bartlett Publishers; 1999: chap 9.

ADDITIONAL RESOURCES

Alexander JM, Grant AM, Campbell MJ. Randomized controlled trial of breast shells and Hoffman's exercises for inverted and non-protractile nipples. *Br Med J.* 1992;304:1030-1032.

Armstrong HC. Techniques of feeding infants: the case for cup feeding. *Res Action.* June 1998;8.

Arnold LDW, Ed. *Recommendations for Collection, Storage, and Handling of a Mother's Milk for her own Infant in the Hospital Setting.* Sandwich MA: Human Milk Banking Association of North America; November 1993.

Arnold LDW, Tully MR, eds. *Guidelines for the Establishment and Operation of A Donor Human Milk Bank.* Sandwich MA: Human Milk Banking Association of North America; 1998.

Auerbach K. *Breastfeeding Techniques and Devices.* Wayne, NJ: Avery Publishing Group; 1985: Lactation Consultant Series, Unit 17.

Auerbach KG. The effect of nipple shields on maternal milk volume. *JOGNN.* 1990;19(5):419-427.

Auerbach, KG. Sequential and simultaneous breastpumping: a comparison. *Intl J Nurs Studies.* 1990;27:257-265.

Barros FC, Victoria CG, Semer TC, et al. Use of pacifiers is associated with decreased breastfeeding duration. *Pediatrics.* 1995;95:497-499.

Blackman JA, Nelson CLA. Reinstituting oral feedings in children fed by gastrostomy tube. *Clin Pediatr.* 1985;34(8):434-438.

Bodley V, et al. Long-term nipple shield use—a positive perspective. *J Hum Lact.* Dec 1996;12(4):301-304.

Brigham M. Mothers' reports of the outcome of nipple shield use. *J Hum Lact.* Dec 1996;12(4):291-297.

Campos RG. Soothing pain-elicited distress in infants with swaddling and pacifiers. *Child Dev.* 1989;60(4):781-792.

Clum D, et al. Use of a silicone nipple shield with premature infants. *J Hum Lact.* 1996;12(4):287-290.

Coreil J, Murphy JE. Maternal commitment, lactation practices, and breast-feeding duration. *JOGNN.* 1988;17:273-278.

Davis HV, Sears RR, Miller, HC, Brodbeck AJ. Effects of cup, bottle and breastfeeding on oral activities of newborn infants. *Pediatrics.* 1948;2:549-555.

Davis, DK, Bell, P. Infant feeding practice and occlusal outcomes. A longitudinal study. *Can Dent Assoc.* 1991;57(7):593-594.

De Coopman JM. *Breastfeeding Management for Health Care Professionals.* Wyandotte, MI: self-published; 1993.

Engebretson JC, Wardell DW. Development of a pacifier for low-birth-weight infants' non-nutritive sucking. *JOGNN.* 1997;26:660-664.

Fildes, Valerie. *Breasts, Bottles And Babies: A History Of Infant Feeding.* Edinburgh: Edinburgh University Press; 1986.

Fildes, Valerie. *Wet Nursing: A History From Antiquity To The Present.* New York: Basil Blackwell; 1988.

Fredeen RC. Cup-feeding of newborn infants. *Pediatrics.* 1948;2:544-548.

Gale CR, Martyn CN. Breastfeeding, dummy use, and adult intelligence. *Lancet.* 1996;347:1072-1075.

Gale Mobbs EJ. Human imprinting and breastfeeding—are the textbooks deficient? *Breastfeed Rev.* 1989;1(14):39-41.

Griffiths RJ. Breast pads: their effectiveness and use by lactating women. *J Hum Lact.* 1993;9(1):19-26.

Healow LK. Finger-feeding a premie. *Midwife Today Childbirth Ed.* 1995; 33:9.

Hunziker UA, Barr RG. Increased carrying reduces infant crying: a randomized controlled trial. *Pediatrics.* 1986;77:641-648.

IBFAN Africa. IBFAN Statement on Cups. *IBFAN Africa News.* June 1986.

Kimble, Claudia. Nonnutritive sucking: adaptation and health for the neonate. *Neonatal Network.* March 1992;11(2):29-33.

Kleinman RE, ed. *Pediatric Nutrition Handbook.* 4th ed. Elk Grove Village IL: American Academy of Pediatrics; 1998.

Kuehl, J. Cup feeding the newborn: what you should know. *J Perinat Neonat Nurs.* 1997;11(2):56-60.

Kurokawa, J. Finger-feeding a premie. *Midwife Today Childbirth Ed.* 1994; 29:39.

Lang S, Lawrence CJ, Orme R Lt. Cup-feeding: an alternative method of infant feeding. *Arch Dis Child.* 1994;71:365-269.

Lang, S. Cup-feeding: an alternative method. *Midwives Chron.* 1994;107: 171-176.

Ludington-Hoe SM, Golant SK. *Kangaroo Care: the Best You Can Do to Help Your Preterm Infant.* New York: Bantam Books; 1993.

Marmet C, Shell E. Training neonates to suck correctly. *Am J Maternal Child Nurs.* 1984;9:401-407.

Marmet C, Shell E. *Lactation Forms: A Guide to Lactation Consultant Charting.* Encino, CA: Lactation Institute; 1993.

Mathur GP, Mathus S, Khanduja GS. Non-nutritive suckling and use of pacifiers. *Indian Pediatr.* Nov 1990;27(11):1187-1189.

McBride M, and Danner S. Sucking disorders in neurologically impaired infants: assessment and facilitation of breastfeeding. *Clin Perinatol.* 12; 1:109-130, 1987.

Measel CP, and Anderson GC. Nonnutritive sucking during tube feedings: effect on clinical course in premature infants, *JOGN Nurs.* Sept-Oct 1979; 8(5):265-272.

Meier P, Anderson GC. Responses of small preterm infants to bottle- and breastfeeding. *MCN.* Mar/Apr 1987;12:97-103.

Meier P. Bottle- and breastfeeding: effects on transcutaneous oxygen pressure and temperature in preterm infants. *Nurs Res.* 1988;37(1):36-41.

Melsen B, et al. Sucking habits and their influence on swallowing pattern and prevalence of malocclusion. *European J Ortho.* 1979;1(4):271-280.

Meyer Palmer M, Crawley K, Bianco IA. Neonatal oral-motor assessment scale: a reliability study. *J Perinat.* 1993;XIII(1):28-35.

Meyer Palmer M, Heyman MB. Assessment and treatment of sensory-versus motor-based feeding problems in very young children. *Inf Young Child.* 1993;6(2):67-73.

Minchin, MK. Positioning for breastfeeding. *Birth.* Jun 1989;16(2):67-79.

Montagu, Ashley. *Touching: the Human Significance of the Skin.* 3rd ed. New York: Harper & Row; 1986.

Morris S, Meyer Palmer M. *The normal acquisition of oral feeding skills: implications for assessment and treatment.* New York: Therapeutic Media; 1982:chaps 2-5.

Narayanan I, Mehta, Dhoudhury DK, Jain BK. Sucking on the emptied breast: non-nutritive sucking with a difference. *Arch Dis Child.* 1991; 66(2):241-244.

Neifert M, Lawrence R, Seacat J. Nipple confusion: toward a formal definition. *J Pediatr.* 1995;126:125-129.

Newman, J. Breastfeeding problems associated with the early introduction of bottles and pacifiers. *J Human Lact.* 1990;6(2):59-63.

Nicholson WL. The use of nipple shields by breastfeeding women. *J Aust Coll Midwives.* June 1993;6(2):18-24.

Niemala M, Uhari M, Mottonen M. A pacifier increases the risk of recurrent otitis media in children in day care centers. *Pediatrics.* 1995;96:884-888.

Novak AJ, Smith WL, Erenberg A. Imaging evaluation of artificial nipples during bottle feeding. *Arch Ped Adoles Med.* 1994;148:40-42.

Nylander G, Lindeman R, Helsing E, Bendvold E. Unsupplemented breastfeeding in the maternity ward. Positive long-term effects. *Acta Obste Gynecol Scand.* 1991;70(3):205-209.

Palmer MM, Crawley K, Bianco IA. Neonatal oral-motor assessment scale: a reliability study, *J Perinatol.* 1993;XIII(1):28-35.

Pottenger FM, Krohn B. Influence of breastfeeding on facial development. *Arch Pediatr.* 1950;57:454-461.

Pryor K, Pryor G. *Nursing Your Baby.* rev ed. New York: Pocket Books; 1991.

Ramsay M, Gisel EG. Neonatal sucking and maternal feeding practices. *Dev Med Child Neurol.* Jan 1996;38(1):34-47.

Renfew M, Fisher C, Arms S. *Bestfeeding: Getting Breastfeeding Right for You.* Berkeley, CA: Celestial Arts; 1990.

Righard L, Alade MO. Breastfeeding and the use of pacifiers. *Birth.* June 1997;24:2.

Righard L, Alade MO. Sucking technique and its effect on success of breastfeeding. *Birth.* December 1992;19:4.

Righard L, Alade MO. Effect of delivery room routines on success of first breastfeed. *Lancet.* 1990;336:1105-1107.

Righard L. Are breastfeeding problems related to incorrect breastfeeding technique and the use of pacifiers and bottles? *Birth.* Mar 1998;25(1): 40-44.

Ross, MW. *Back to the breast: retraining infant suckling patterns.* Schaumburg IL. La Leche League International; 1987: Lactation Consultant Series, Unit 15.

Smith W., et al. Physiology of sucking in the normal term infant using real-time ultrasound. *Radiology.* 1985;156:379.

Tappero EP, Honeyfield ME. *Physical Assessment of the Newborn.* Petaluma, CA: NICU Ink; 1993.

Taylor PM, Maloni JA, Brown DR. Early suckling and prolonged breastfeeding. *Am J Dis Child.* Feb 1986;140(2):151-154.

Thorley V. Cup-feeding: problems created by incorrect use. *J Hum Lact.* 1997;12:54-55.

Trenouth MN, Campbell AN. Questionnaire evaluation of feeding methods for cleft lip and palate neonates. *Int J Paediatr Dent.* 1996;6(4): 241-244.

Victora CG, Tomaje E, Olinto, MTA, Barros FC. Use of pacifiers and breastfeeding duration. *Lancet.* 1993;341:404-406.

Victora, CG, Behague DP, Barros FC, Olinto MTA, Weiderpass E. Pacifier use and short breastfeeding duration: cause, consequence or coincidence? *Pediatrics.* 1997;99:445-453.

Weber F, et al. An ultrasonographic study of the organization of sucking and swallowing by newborn infants. *Dev Med Child Neurol.* 1986;28:19-24.

Widstrom AM, Thingstrom-Paulsson J. The position of the tongue during rooting reflexes elicited in newborn infants before the first suckle. *Acta Paediatr Scand.* 1993;82:281-283.

Wiessinger D. A breastfeeding teaching tool using a sandwich analogy for latch-on. *J Hum Lact.* Mar 1998;14(1):51-56.

Wilson JM, Ed. *Oral-motor function and dysfunction in children.* University of North Carolina at Chapel Hill; 1977:Section 1; section 2, chap 2.

Wilson-Clay B. Clinical use of silicone nipple shields. *J Hum Lact.* Dec 1996;12(4):279-285.

Wolf LS, Glass RP. *Feeding and Swallowing Disorders in Infancy.* San Antonio, TX: Therapy Skill Builders; 1992.

Woolridge MW, Baum JD, Drewett RF. Effect of a traditional and of a new nipple shield on sucking patterns and milk flow. *Early Hum Dev.* 1980; 4:357-364.

Woolridge M. Anatomy of infant sucking. *Midwifery.* 1986;2:164-171.

12 Techniques

In the exam blueprint, 19 to 33 questions are dedicated to techniques, specifically: positioning, latch, and management skills; normal feeding patterns, milk collection and storage.

SUBTOPICS INCLUDED IN THIS CATEGORY

1. Positioning, latch
2. Management skills
    a. Assessing a breastfeed
        i.   Observing; history
        ii. Assessing infant suck, lactating breast, milk transfer
        iii. Objective tools
    b. Care planning and following-up
    c. Kangaroo care (skin-to-skin care)
3. Normal feeding patterns
4. Infant state
5. Milk collection and storage

CORE READING

Black RF, Jarman L, Simpson J. *Lactation Specialist Self-Study Modules #1-4.* Sudbury, MA: Jones & Bartlett Publishers; 1998: module 2, chap 1A, B, C; chap 3A.

Frantz K. *Breastfeeding Product Guide.* Sunland CA: Geddes Productions; 1994.

Lauwers J, Shinskie D. *Counseling the Nursing Mother.* 3rd ed. Sudbury, MA: Jones & Bartlett Publishers; 2000: chaps 10, 19.

Lawrence RA, Lawrence RM. *Breastfeeding a Guide for the Medical Profession.* 5th ed. St. Louis: Mosby; 1999: chap 8, 13, 20: appendices G, H.

Morbacher N, Stock J. *the Breastfeeding Answer Book.* rev ed. Schaumburg, IL: La Leche League International, 1997: chaps 3, 4, 8, 9.

Riordan J, Auerbach KG. *Breastfeeding and Human Lactation,* 2nd ed. Sudbury, MA: Jones & Bartlett Publishers; 1999: chap 9.

ADDITIONAL RESOURCES

_____. *The Womanly Art of Breastfeeding.* 6th rev ed. Schaumburg, IL: La Leche League International; 1997.

AAP workgroup on Breastfeeding. Breastfeeding and the Use of Human Milk. *Pediatrics.* 1997;100(6):1035-1039.

Akre J, ed. *Infant Feeding, The Physiological Basis.* Bulletin of the World Health Organization Supplement to Vol. 67 (1989) Geneva: World Health Organization; 1991.

Alexander JM, Grant AM, Campbell MJ. Randomized controlled trial of breast shells and Hoffman's exercises for inverted and non-protractile nipples. *Br Med J.* 1992;304:1030-1032.

Armstrong, HC. Techniques of feeding infants: the case for cup feeding. *Res Action.* 1998;8.

Arnold LDW, ed. *Recommendations for Collection, Storage, and Handling of a Mother's Milk for her own Infant in the Hospital Setting.* Sandwich MA: Human Milk Banking Association of North America; 1993.

Arnold LDW, Tully MR, Eds. *Guidelines for the Establishment and Operation of A Donor Human Milk Bank.* Sandwich MA: Human Milk Banking Association of North America; 1998.

Auerbach K. *Breastfeeding Techniques and Devices.* Wayne, NJ: Avery Publishing Group; 1985: Lactation Consultant Series, Unit 17.

Bumgarner NJ. *Mothering Your Nursing Toddler.* Revised Ed. Schaumburg, IL: LaLeche League International; 2000.

Butte NF, Wills C, Jean CA, Smith EO, Garza C. Feeding patterns of exclusively breastfed infants during the first four months of life. *Early Hum Dev.* 1985;12(3):291-300.

Casey CE, Neifert MR, Seacat JM, Neville MC. Nutrient intake by breastfed infants during the first five days after birth. *Am J Dis Child.* 1986; 140(9):933-936.

De Coopman JM. *Breastfeeding Management for Health Care Professionals.* Wyandotte, MI: self-published; 1993.

DeCarvalho M, Robertson S, Friedman A, Klaus M. Effect of frequent breastfeeding on early milk production and infant weight gain. *Pediatrics.* 1983;72(3):307-311.

DeCarvalho M, Robertson S, Merkatz R, Klaus M. Milk intake and frequency of feeding in breastfed infants. *Early Hum Dev.* 1982;7(2): 155-163.

DeMarzo S, Seacat J, Neifert M. Initial weight loss and return to birth weight criteria for breastfed infants: challenging the rules of thumb. *AJDC.* 1991;145:402.

Desmarais L, Browne S. *Inadequate weight gain in breastfeeding infants: Assessments and resolution.* Schaumburg, IL: La Leche League International; 1990: Lactation Consultant Series, Unit 8.

Dettwyler K, Fishman. Infant feeding practices and growth. *Ann Rev Anthro.* 1992;21:171-204.

Dubignon J, Cooper D. Good and poor feeding behavior in the neonatal period. *Infant Behav Dev.* 1980;3:395-408.

Elias MF, Nicolson NA, Bora C, Johnston J. Sleep/wake patterns of breastfed infants in the first 2 years of life. *Pediatrics.* 1986;77:322-329.

Foman SJ. *Nutrition of Normal Infants,* St. Louis: Mosby; 1993.

Fomon SJ, Filer Jr LJ, Anderson TA, Ziegler EE. Recommendations for feeding normal infants. *Pediatrics.* 1979;63(1):52-59.

Guidelines for the establishment and operation of a donor human milk bank. Sandwich MA: Human Milk Banking Association of North America; 1994.

Hamosh M, Ellis LA, Pollock DR, Henderson TR, Hamosh P. Breastfeeding and the working mother: effect of time and temperature of short-term storage on proteolysis, lipolysis, and bacteria growth in milk. *Pediatrics.* 1996;97(4):492-498.

Healow LK. Finger-feeding a premie. *Midwif Today Childbirth Ed.* 1995; 33:9.

Heinig MH, Nommsen LA, Peerson MH, Lonnerdal B, Dewey KG. Energy and protein intakes of breastfed and formula-fed infants during the first year of life and their association with growth velocity: the DARLING study. *Am J Clin Nutr.* 1993;58:152-161.

Hendricks KM. Weaning recommendations: the scientific basis. *Nutr Rev.* 1992;50(5):125-133.

Howie PW, Houston MJ, Cook A, Smart L, McArdle T, McNeilly AS. How long should a breastfeed last? *Early Hum Dev.* 1981;5(1):71-77.

International Lactation Consultant Association: *Position Paper on Infant Feeding.* Raleigh, NC: ILCA; 1994.

Jocson MA, Mason EO, Schanler RJ. The effects of nutrient fortification and varying storage conditions on host defense properties of human milk. *Pediatrics.* 1997;100:240-243.

Kuehl, J. Cup feeding the newborn: what you should know. *J Perinat Neonat Nurs.* 1997;11(2):56-60.

Kurokawa, J. Finger-feeding a premie. *Midwife Today Childbirth Ed.* 1994; 29:39.

Lang S, Lawrence CJ, Orme R Lt. Cup-feeding: an alternative method of infant feeding. *Arch Dis Child.* 1994;71:365-69.

Lang, S. Cup-feeding: an alternative method. *Midwives Chron.* 1994;107: 171-176.

Marmet C, Shell E. Training neonates to suck correctly. *Am J Maternal Child Nurs.* 1984;9:401-407.

Matheney RJ, Birch LL, Picciano MF. Control of intake by human-milk-fed infants: relationship between feeding size and interval. *Dev Psychobiol.* 1990;23(6):511-518.

McKenna JJ, Mosko SS, Dungy C, McAninch J. Sleep and arousal patterns of co-sleeping human mother/infant pairs: a preliminary physiological study with implications for the study of sudden infant death syndrome (SIDS) *Am J Phys Anthropol.* 1990;83(3):331-347.

McKenna JJ, Mosko SS, Richard CA. Bedsharing promotes breastfeeding. *Pediatrics.* 1997;100(2 pt 1):214-219.

McKenna JJ, Mosko SS. Sleep and arousal, synchrony and independence, among mothers and infants sleeping apart and together (same bed): an experiment in evolutionary medicine. *Acta Paediatr Suppl.* 1994;397: 94-102.

McKenna JJ, Thoman EB, Anders TF, Sadeh A, Schectman VL, Glotzbach SF. Pediatric review: infant-parent co-sleeping in an evolutionary perspective: implications for understanding infant sleep development and the sudden infant death syndrome. *Sleep.* 1993;16(3):263-282.

Meier P, Anderson GC. Responses of small preterm infants to bottle- and breastfeeding. *MCN.* 1987;12:97-103.

Meier P. Bottle- and breastfeeding: effects on transcutaneous oxygen pressure and temperature in preterm infants. *Nurs Res.* 1988;37(1):36-41.

Meyer Palmer M, Crawley K, Bianco IA. Neonatal oral-motor assessment scale: a reliability study. *J Perinat.* 1993;XIII(1):28-35.

Minchin, MK. Positioning for breastfeeding. *Birth.* 1989;16(2):67-79.

Montagu, A. *Touching: the Human Significance of the Skin.* 3rd ed. New York: Harper & Row; 1986.

Morris S, Meyer Palmer M, ed. *The normal acquisition of oral feeding skills: implications for assessment and treatment.* New York: Therapeutic Media; 1982: chaps 2-5.

Narayanan I, Mehta, Dhoudhury DK, Jain BK. Sucking on the emptied breast: non-nutritive sucking with a difference. *Arch Dis Child.* 1991; 66(2):241-244.

Neifert M, Lawrence R, Seacat J. Nipple confusion: toward a formal definition. *J Pediatr.* 1995;126:125-129.

Neifert MR. The optimization of breastfeeding in the perinatal period. *Clin Perinatol.* 1998;25(2):303-326.

Nylander G, Lindemann R, Helsing E, Bendvoid E. Unsupplemented breastfeeding in the maternity ward. Positive long-term effects. *Acta Obstet Gynecol Scand.* 1991;70(3):205-209.

Palmer MM, Crawley K, Bianco IA. Neonatal oral-motor assessment scale: a reliability study. *J Perinatol.* 1993;XIII(1):28-35.

Paul K, Dittrichova J, Papousek H. Infant feeding behavior: development in patterns and motivation. *Devel Psychobiol.* 1996;29(7):563-576.

Quillin SI. Infant and mother sleep patterns during 4th postpartum week. *Issues Compr Pediatr Nurs.* 1997;20(2):115-123.

Ramsay M, Gisel EG. Neonatal sucking and maternal feeding practices. *Dev Med Child Neurol.* 1996;38(1):34-47.

Renfew M, Fisher C, Arms S. *Bestfeeding: Getting Breastfeeding Right for You.* Berkeley, CA: Celestial Arts; 1990.

Righard L, Alade MO. Effect of delivery room routines on success of first breastfeed. *Lancet.* 1990;336:1105-1107.

Ross, MW. *Back to the breast: retraining infant suckling patterns.* Schaumburg, IL: La Leche League International; 1987: Lactation Consultant Series, Unit 15.

Satter E. *Child of Mine: Feeding with Love and Good Sense.* Palo Alto, CA: Bull Publishing; 1983.

Savage F. *Helping Mothers to Breastfeed.* Nairobi, Kenya: African Medical and Research Foundation; 1994.

Smith W, et al. Physiology of sucking in the normal term infant using real-time ultrasound. *Radiology.* 1985;156:379.

Stuart-Macadam P, Dettwyler KA. *Breastfeeding: Biocultural Perspectives.* New York: Aldine De Gruyter; 1995.

Taylor PM, Maloni JA, Brown DR. Early suckling and prolonged breastfeeding. *Am J Dis Child.* 1986;140(2):151-154.

Widstrom AM, Thingstrom-Paulsson J. The position of the tongue during rooting reflexes elicited in newborn infants before the first suckle. *Acta Paediatr Scand.* 1993;82:281-283.

Wiessinger D. A breastfeeding teaching tool using a sandwich analogy for latch-on. *J Hum Lact.* 1998;14(1):51-56.

Wolf LS, Glass RP. *Feeding and Swallowing Disorders in Infancy.* San Antonio, TX: Therapy Skill Builders; 1992.

Woolridge, M. Anatomy of infant suckling. *Midwifery.* 1986;2:164-171.

Wright P. Learning experiences in feeding behaviour during infancy. *J Psychosom Res.* 1988;32(6):613-619.

Yamauchi Y, Yamanouchi I. Breastfeeding frequency during the first 24 hours after birth in full-term neonates. *Pediatrics* Aug 1990;86(2): 171-175.

13

Public Health and Advocacy

In the exam blueprint, 4 to 8 questions are dedicated to public health and advocacy, specifically: community education; creating and implementing clinical and research protocols: WHO Code, Baby Friendly Hospital Initiative implementation; skills; interaction with policy makers.

SUBTOPICS INCLUDED IN THIS CATEGORY

1. Community education; vulnerable populations
2. Creating and implementing clinical and research protocols
3. WHO Code; other international documents, conferences, and initiatives
4. Baby Friendly Hospital Initiative implementation
5. Skills (advocacy)
6. Interaction with policy makers; changing public policy

CORE READING

_____. *Protecting, Promoting and Supporting Breastfeeding: The Special Role of Maternity Services.* A Joint WHO/UNICEF Statement. Geneva: World Health Organization Nutrition Unit; 1989.

Black RF, Jarman L, Simpson J. *Lactation Specialist Self-Study Modules #1-4.* Sudbury, MA: Jones & Bartlett Publishers; 1998: module 1, chap 3 A & B.

Lauwers J, Shinskie D. *Counseling the Nursing Mother.* 3rd ed. Sudbury, MA: Jones & Bartlett Publishers; 2000: chaps 1, 9, 26, appendix on resources.

Lawrence RA, Lawrence RM. *Breastfeeding, a Guide for the Medical Profession.* 5th ed. St Louis: Mosby; 1999: chap 1, 2, 13, 21, 22 appendices K, L, M.

Riordan J, Auerbach KG. *Breastfeeding and Human Lactation.* 2nd ed. Sudbury, MA: Jones & Bartlett Publishers; 1999: chaps 1, 8, appendices B, C, E, F.

ADDITIONAL RESOURCES

American Academy of Pediatrics Work Group on Breastfeeding, 1997. Breastfeeding and the use of human milk. *Pediatrics.* 1997;100:1035-1039. (Policy # RE9729).

Auerbach KG. Breastfeeding promotion: why it doesn't work. *J Human Lact.* 1990;6(2):45-46.

Baby Milk: Destruction of a world resource. London: Catholic Institute for International Relations; 1993.

Baumslag N, Michels D. *Milk, Money and Madness.* Westport CT: Bergin & Garvey; 1995.

Breaking the Rules, Stretching the Rules 1998: A worldwide report on violations of the WHO/UNICEF International Code of Marketing of Breastmilk Substitutes. Penang, Malaysia; 1998.

Breastfeeding Advocacy Kit. Weston MA: National Alliance for Breastfeeding Advocacy; 1997.

Breastfeeding in the First Week: A counseling guide for health care professionals. Des Moines, IA: Iowa Department of Public Health; 1998.

Breastfeeding Saves Lives: the impact of breastfeeding in infant survival. Washington DC: NURTURE and the Institute for Reproductive Health; 1996.

Breastfeeding: The Technical Basis And Recommendations For Action. Geneva: World Health Organization; 1993.

Cadwell K. *Growing the Breastfeeding Friendly Community.* Weston MA: National Alliance for Breastfeeding Advocacy; 1996.

Chalmers I. Minimizing harm and maximizing benefit during innovation in health care: controlled or uncontrolled experiment? *Birth.* 1986;13(3): 155-164.

Davis M. *The Lactation Consultant's Clinical Practice Manual.* Dayton, OH: Bright Future Lactation Resource Centre; 1998.

Greiner, T. Infant Feeding Policy Options for Governments. *Report for Infant Feeding Consortium.* Ithaca, NY: Cornell University Program on International Nutrition; 1982.

Hauth J, Merenstein GB, eds: *Guidelines for Perinatal Care.* 4th ed. Elk Grove Village, IL: American Academy of Pediatrics; Washington DC: American College of Obstetricians and Gynecologists; 1997.

Institute of Medicine (Subcommittee on Nutrition during Lactation, Food and Nutrition Board). *Nutrition during Lactation.* Washington DC: National Academy of Sciences; 1991.

Institute of Medicine. *Nutrition during Pregnancy.* Washington DC: National Academy of Sciences; 1991.

Koop CE. *Report of the Surgeon General's Workshop on Breastfeeding and Human Lactation.* Washington DC: DHHS Publication # HRS-D-MC-84-2; 1984.

Kyenkya-Isabrrye M. UNICEF launches the Baby-Friendly Hospital Initiative. *Am J Maternal Child Nurs.* 1990;17:177-179.

Lawrence R. *A Review of the Medical Benefits and Contraindications to Breastfeeding in the United States* (Maternal and Child Health Technical Information Bulletin). Arlington VA: National Center for Education in Maternal and Child Health; October 1997.

Palmer G. *The Politics of Breastfeeding.* 2nd ed. London: Pandora Press; 1993.

Salisbury L, Blackwell AG. *An Administrative Petition To The United States Food And Drug Administration And Department Of Health And Human Services.* San Francisco CA: Public Advocates; 1981.

Sharbaugh CS. *Call to Action: Better Nutrition for Mothers, Children, And Families.* Washington DC: National Center for Education in Maternal and Child Health; 1990.

Smith LJ. A score sheet for evaluating breastfeeding educational materials. *J Hum Lact.* 1995;11:3-7-311.

Smith LJ. *Adequate Breastfeeding Care in the United States: A Theoretical and Practical Guide to Breastfeeding Support.* Dayton, OH: Bright Future Lactation Resource Centre; 1997.

Sterken E. Role of the World Health Organization in the promotion of breastfeeding. *Can Fam Physician.* 1990;36:1546-1550.

The Progress of Nations 1998. New York: United Nations Children's Fund; 1998.

The State of the World's Children 1998. New York: United Nation Children's Fund; 1998.

U.S. Committee for UNICEF. *Annual Report 1996-1997.* New York: United Nations Children's Fund; 1997.

UNICEF Annual Report 1998. New York: United Nations Children's Fund; 1998.

US Department of Health and Human Services Public Health Service. *Healthy People 2000: National Promotion and Disease Prevention Objectives.* Washington DC: National Center for Education in Maternal and Child Health; 1991.

US Department of Health and Human Services Public Health Service. *Healthy People 2000: National Promotion and Disease Prevention Objectives.* Washington DC: National Center for Education in Maternal and Child Health; 1991.

Van Esterik, P. *Beyond the Breast-Bottle Controversy.* New Brunswick NJ: Rutgers University Press; 1989.

Waggett GG, Waggett RR. Breast is best: legislation supporting is an absolute bare necessity—a model approach. *Maryland J Contemp Legal Issues.* 1995;6(1).

14

Introduction to the Practice Tests

PREPARING FOR THE PRACTICE EXAMS

Exam Structure

1. Each item (test question) has an introductory sentence or paragraph (stem). All the information necessary to answer the question is given in the stem and/or the response choices. *Assume there are no additional complicating circumstances.* Do not read more into the question than is provided, and don't waste time asking "but what if." Each question is testing only ONE concept.

2. Items 121 through 200 also require viewing of a picture or diagram in order to answer the question. Look for the obvious—what you need to see will be clearly visible, even if there are extraneous features visible in the picture.

3. Some items refer to situations involving a mother and/or baby and ask what "you" should do. The "you" refers to your role as a lactation consultant. If you have another professional role, which authorizes you to perform additional functions (such as medical diagnosis or prescribing medications), do not include these functions in the role of the lactation consultant for the purposes of this exam.

4. Each item ends with a specific question, which should be read carefully to know what is being asked. A key word may be capitalized, such as "the MOST appropriate action" or "your FIRST response." These represent the types of decisions that frequently occur in lactation consultant practice. For example, the lactation consultant may need to know which intervention is the MOST likely or LEAST likely to be helpful or effective.

5. Some questions will ask for the MOST (or LEAST) likely cause or explanation for a situation. These test knowledge of the general principles of clinical practice. Still others will present several interventions, asking

which should be suggested FIRST. These are designed to test the lactation consultant's attitudes and skill.

6. There is ONE correct answer for each question. Common misconceptions and outdated ideas are often used as incorrect responses.

7. The items selected for the practice exams come from a large "pool" of possible questions, which is modeled after IBLCE's large data pool. Therefore you may find a few questions repeated on more than one exam.

8. Gender pronouns: The mother, obviously, is always referred to with female pronouns. Where a sample question refers to a specific baby, such as in a photograph, the matching gender pronouns are used. For questions simply referring to "a baby," I've tried to alternate between male and female pronouns rather randomly, and any overemphasis on one gender is accidental.

9. There is no penalty for guessing. If you can eliminate one or two choices as clearly wrong, but can't decide between the remaining choices, take a guess—you have a 50% chance of being right.

Taking the Practice Exams

> *Disclaimer:* To the best of my knowledge, I have closely approximated the difficulty, type of questions, and overall approach used by the IBLCE. Although I was intimately involved in developing the original (1985) exam blueprint and examination, I have not had access to the IBLCE examination content for several years. *The questions in this book have never been submitted to the IBLCE.*
>
> **Passing this exam simulation should not be construed to be a guarantee of passing the IBLCE examination.**

Instructions

There are three different exams, each with unique questions. Start with any one of the sample exams. Take the exam, analyze your results, then focus further study on any areas of weakness.

Answer all the questions. Each question has one and only one correct answer. No partial credit is given. There is no penalty for guessing. *Use the answer sheets provided.* Be sure to darken (fill in) the appropriate circle for each item on the answer sheets.

Part 1.   This part contains 120 multiple-choice questions. Allow up to 3 hours to complete this section. Take a break of 30 minutes or more before beginning Part 2.

Part 2.   This part contains 80 multiple-choice questions utilizing clinical photographs. **The clinical photographs are on the enclosed CD-ROM.** Look at the corresponding picture for *each* question to answer these test items. Everything you need to see to answer the question is clearly visible. Allow up to 2 hours to complete this section.

The Answer Keys begin on page 199. The answer key includes the correct answer; an explanation or rationale; the discipline and period, whether knowledge or application; and the degree of difficulty. Degree of difficulty is calculated by how closely the wrong answers approximate the correct answer. The easiest questions are rated 2; the most difficult are rated 5.

Scoring

The passing grade for the practice exams is 65%, or 130 correct answers out of 200 questions. All 200 questions are scored as one complete exam. To analyze your individual areas of strength and weakness, examine the disciplines and periods for each question to identify patterns.

   If you disagree with an answer, reread about that topic in several of the resources, talk with experienced lactation consultants, and carefully examine the incorrect answers. On the actual IBLCE examinations each year, poorly performing questions are always identified and removed before the final scoring. There is no mechanism for following this practice with this book.

TO FURTHER PREPARE FOR THE IBLCE EXAMINATION

Consider Using These Proven Successful Strategies

☐ Review your knowledge and skills about 2 to 3 days before the exam. Then put away all books and references until after the exam. Cramming does not help and increases anxiety.

☐ Do something relaxing and enjoyable on the 2 days prior to the test. Get some fresh air and a change of pace on the day before the test.

☐ Allow sufficient travel time to avoid feeling rushed. Get a good night's sleep, and follow your normal routine as closely as possible. Wear comfortable clothes in layers.

☐ Eat normally and emphasize protein-rich foods that will help you stay alert and focused. Drink water, which facilitates brain and nerve function.

Trust yourself

Give yourself positive affirmations and trust your knowledge of mothers and babies; for example, "I know how to help breastfeeding mothers and babies." "I am a good test taker." Use calming/centering techniques that have served you well in the past, such as taking a deep breath, closing your eyes, meditating, or focusing on your breathing. Visualize recalling all the wealth of your knowledge, passing the exam, and receiving your excellent score report. Anxiety isn't always a bad thing. Allow yourself to feel any anxiety that arises—it will pass, just as a labor contraction does, and you will feel normal afterward. A slight rise in adrenal hormones may sharpen your focus and concentration, even as the same hormones have the unpleasant side effect of making you feel "testy."

Carefully Examine Each Question Before Answering

Read each question, especially the stem, very carefully before you answer. *Never* change an answer unless you are absolutely, positively *sure* the first answer was clearly wrong. If you are unsure, rely on your best guess and first hunch. Allow yourself to miss a few questions. Review the *Candidate's Guide* one more time, paying attention to the structure and format of test items.

Be Patient and Calm while you Wait for the Exam Results

At lunch and after the exam, resist the temptation to discuss your answers with other candidates. This is a sure recipe for self-doubt and increased anxiety! Remember that you only have to *pass*. Nobody has ever scored 100% in the entire history of the exam. If the worst happens and you don't get a passing grade, you can take the exam again in subsequent years. Use your score report to focus on areas of weakness. Take additional formal and informal educational courses, arrange mentoring experiences, and use the time to reflect on long-term goals and aspirations.

Keep reading to stay up to date, whether or not you pass the exam. New information is constantly appearing that will either confirm or change existing practices. Avail yourself of as many resources as possible, especially texts and reference books. It's wise to budget for several new books and at least one major breastfeeding conference each year. Attend continuing educational programs in breastfeeding and related fields. Read the *Journal of Human Lactation.* Search the Internet frequently for pertinent information.

Use your new credential proudly! Join ILCA and local coalitions or affiliate groups and participate as time allows. Continue building a support network for yourself as a lactation consultant. Just like the mothers you work with, lactation consultants need a support system, too!

A BRIEF HISTORY OF THE IBLCE EXAM

The first exam was held simultaneously in Washington, DC and Melbourne, Australia in 1985. It was the first health credentialing examination to begin internationally, not just nationally or regionally.

The Task Analysis done prior to the examination analyzes the issues and problems known to affect breastfeeding. Those concepts, topics, and problems that are most *critical* to the mother's ability to breastfeed and that occur most *frequently* will appear in higher concentration than those issues that are either less critical, occur less frequently, or both. The most recent worldwide survey (1998-1999) results were used in determining the current blueprint. Surveys are conducted every 5 years, and the distribution of questions is adjusted accordingly shortly thereafter. Each survey to date has resulted in a slight redistribution of questions in the various disciplines and stages.

The requirement of a 4-year college degree for Pathway A began in 1988; other pathways were subsequently added to reflect alternate means of preparation. The pass-fail score is adjusted yearly, based on the relative difficulty of the exam as determined by the Exam Committee and the psychometrician. Therefore the exact passing score is not the same every year. The mean passing score for all years to date is 64%. Because of the rigorous prerequisites, the exam has a very high pass rate of 92%. The average (mean) score for all years is 73%. In most years, a score in the mid to high 80s falls in the top 5% of candidates. The highest score ever earned (as of this writing) is 93%.

IBLCE identifies weak areas every year. These have included infant growth and development, statistics and research, maternal-infant cosleeping, ethical and legal issues, HIV, maternal and infant anatomy, immunology and infectious disease, and public health. The stages of prematurity, 4-6 months, and 7-12 months often are problematic for many candidates. Picture questions are better discriminators than the word questions, meaning that the stronger candidates perform even better on the picture section while the weaker candidates are even weaker on the picture questions. The number of picture questions has gradually increased over the years.

After initial scoring, the exam committee analyzes every test question and discards several that performed poorly (failed to discriminate between the candidates). The exam is then rescored and the results sent to the candidates. Each candidate receives a score report, which includes a breakdown of their performance by developmental stage and discipline. In 1999, over 100 sites tested about 2000 candidates. The exam has been translated into at least 8 languages. The IBLCE examination is a highly respected example of evidence-based, globally valid professional credentialing.

GENERAL PURPOSE
NCS®
ANSWER SHEET
form no. 4521

IMPORTANT DIRECTIONS
FOR MARKING ANSWERS

- Use #2 pencil only.
- Do NOT use ink or ballpoint pens.
- Make heavy black marks that fill the circle completely.
- Erase cleanly any answer you wish to change.
- Make no stray marks on the answer sheet.

EXAMPLES

WRONG
1 ① ⊗ ③ ④ ⑤

WRONG
2 ① ② ⊘ ④ ⑤

WRONG
3 ① ② ③ ◑ ⑤

RIGHT
4 ① ② ③ ● ⑤

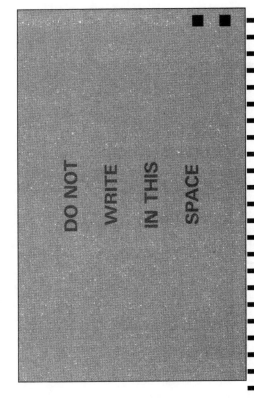

DO NOT WRITE IN THIS SPACE

Trans-Optic® by NCS MPF-4521: 3231302928   Printed in U.S.A.   © 1977 by National Computer Systems, Inc.

81

Exam Questions

1. A woman with a 5-month-old exclusively breastfed baby is pre-scribed amoxicillin for her breast infection. The possible conse-quences for the infant are:
   a. interference with bilirubin binding.
   b. vomiting and dehydration.
   c. none.
   d. diarrhea or loose stools.

2. A laboring woman has received magnesium sulfate with intravenous fluids to control her blood pressure. Her baby is now several hours old and is having trouble breastfeeding. The MOST LIKELY expla-nation for this is:
   a. her breasts are edematous from the magnesium sulfate and IV fluids.
   b. the medication affected the baby's ability to suck.
   c. her milk tastes unpleasant because of the medication.
   d. the drug reduced the amount of colostrum available, and the baby is frustrated.

3. A breastfeeding mother of a 3-week-old baby needs oral surgery for an abscessed tooth. Her dentist is concerned that the antiinflamma-tory drug he plans to prescribe may appear in her milk and cause problems for her baby. Which of the following statements is TRUE?
   a. Antiinflammatory drugs cause severe bleeding in breastfed ba-bies.
   b. Most drugs appear in high concentrations in milk.
   c. Breastfeeding will retard healing of her surgical incision.
   d. Antiinflammatory drugs are generally compatible with breast-feeding.

4. Which drug property results in MORE transfer of the drug into mother's milk?
   a. milk-plasma ratio <1.0
   b. molecular weight >300
   c. high protein binding
   d. lipid solubility

5. A breastfeeding mother is prescribed fluconazole to treat a vaginal infection. She asks the lactation consultant whether it is safe to take this drug while breastfeeding. All of the following are appropriate responses by the lactation consultant EXCEPT:
   a. Yes, it's safe to take fluconazole while breastfeeding.
   b. What has the baby's pediatrician said?
   c. I would be glad to look it up in reference books.
   d. What is your baby's age and health status?

6. The most important determinant of drug penetration into milk is the mother's:
   a. plasma level.
   b. weight.
   c. blood type.
   d. milk storage capacity.

7. A mother was given high doses of pain-relieving drugs during labor. When the baby's cord blood is tested for the presence of drugs, none is found. The MOST LIKELY explanation is:
   a. pain-relieving drugs are lipid soluble and concentrate in the infant brain.
   b. pain-relieving drugs do not cross the placenta.
   c. the mother's body metabolizes most drugs before birth.
   d. pain-relieving drugs have a very short half-life.

8. A newborn baby, 6 hours old, is awake and alert but having trouble breastfeeding. Which of the following is the LEAST likely cause of his difficulty?
   a. Mother received antibiotic treatment for group B streptococcus during labor.
   b. Mother was given epidural anesthesia four hours before delivery.
   c. Mother received narcotic analgesia immediately prior to delivery.
   d. Mother's labor was stimulated by pitocin.

9. When selecting a drug to be given to a breastfeeding woman, which of the following drug properties is MOST IMPORTANT to consider?
   a. absorption from the GI tract
   b. protein binding
   c. milk/plasma ratio
   d. pediatric half-life

10. A ten-hour-old healthy, full-term baby has a blood sugar level of 36 mg/dL (2 mmol/L). The BEST treatment is to:
    a. Ask the mother to breastfeed her baby.
    b. Do nothing.
    c. Give the baby a bottle of glucose water.
    d. Give the baby 30 ml [1 oz] of artificial baby milk.

11. Twenty-seven-year-old Madeleine is having her first baby in three weeks. She asks her health care provider if she will be able to breastfeed after having a breast reduction with her nipple autotransplanted at the age of 19. The BEST response is:
    a. He tells her there will be no problem breastfeeding.
    b. It may be possible for the first 3 months.
    c. She may not be able to breastfeed.
    d. She should try and see what happens.

12. At 14 days postbirth, a mother tells you that she has bright red vaginal bleeding and that her baby (birthweight 9 lbs 2 oz) seems constantly hungry. The MOST LIKELY explanation for this is:
    a. large-for-gestational age baby.
    b. early return of menses.
    c. uterine infection.
    d. retained placenta.

13. Allergy in children is associated with all of the following EXCEPT:
    a. a strong history of allergy in parents.
    b. over half the visits to pediatric practices in the first year of life.
    c. one third of chronic illnesses in children under age 17.
    d. asthma, which accounts for one third of all lost school days.

14. A breastfeeding woman with multiple sclerosis (MS) should be told all of the following EXCEPT:
    a. use extra household help whenever you can.
    b. many medications used for MS are compatible with breastfeeding.
    c. breastfeeding lowers the risk that her baby will develop multiple sclerosis.
    d. breastfeeding decreases the likelihood of acute episodes of MS during the early postpartum period.

15. A breastfeeding mother complains of a lump in her breast. Which characteristic is LEAST likely to be related to lactation?
    a. The lump feels like a soft fluid-filled sac.
    b. The skin over the lump is red and warm.
    c. The mother began running a low-grade fever at the same time the lump appeared.
    d. The lump does not change size before and after the baby feeds.

16. A breastfeeding infant has been diagnosed with oral thrush. You should recommend all of the following interventions EXCEPT:
    a. begin simultaneous treatment of the baby and mother's breast.
    b. unless the mother has signs of infection, treat only the baby's mouth with an antifungal medication.
    c. check mother's nipples for signs or symptoms of infection.
    d. assume that mother's nipples, all infant sucking objects, and possibly other infant areas are infected until proved otherwise.

17. You are asked to evaluate a baby's ability to breastfeed before discharge following an uncomplicated hospital birth 12 hours ago. The baby weighs about 2700 g, or 6 lbs. Which of the following characteristics of her sucking would lead you to suspect that this child was NOT born at term?
    a. moves smoothly from rooting behavior to latch-on
    b. sucks, swallows, and breathes in a coordinated rhythm
    c. sucks in short bursts with pauses
    d. begins by sucking rapidly, then slows to a steady rhythm

18. Which method of family planning is MOST LIKELY to interfere with breastfeeding?
    a. tubal ligation
    b. progestin-only oral contraceptives
    c. cervical cap or diaphragm
    d. natural family planning (periodic abstinence)

19. A mother is concerned that tandem nursing may be harmful to her new baby or older breastfeeding child. Your FIRST response is to:
    a. recommend weaning the older baby.
    b. reassure the mother that tandem breastfeeding is not harmful to either child.
    c. recommend that the mother reduce the time the older child is at the breast.
    d. recommend that she feed the new baby first, before breastfeeding the older baby.

20. The grandmother of a 4-week-old exclusively breastfed baby who has 5 to 6 profuse yellow loose stools every day is worried, and asks for an explanation. The MOST LIKELY cause for stools of this kind is:
    a. diarrhea.
    b. infection with an intestinal parasite.
    c. mother recently ate bright yellow squash.
    d. normal stools.

21. Cholecystokinin, which is released by sucking, has which of the following effects?
    a. arousal
    b. satiety
    c. agitation
    d. depression

22. The husband of a breastfeeding woman is eager for his wife to be as amorous as she was before his son was born three months ago. He asks you for some suggestions that will help her feel more eager for his lovemaking. Your BEST response is:
    a. You'll just have to learn to live with it. When the baby weans, your relationship will get better.
    b. Try helping her with the baby, housework, and cooking. That would probably be considered great "foreplay."
    c. It would be more appropriate for me to talk directly with your wife about this subject.
    d. You may want to use some lubricant, time your lovemaking around the baby's sleep and nursing pattern, and take your time to help her get into the mood.

23. A mother is exclusively breastfeeding her 5-month-old, and her menses have not yet returned. What is her chance of pregnancy?
    a. 7% to 8%
    b. 5% to 6%
    c. 3% to 4%
    d. 1% to 2%

24. Which statement regarding the timing of Lactogenesis II is FALSE?
    a. begins 30 to 40 hours after delivery of the placenta
    b. may initially go unnoticed by mother
    c. may be delayed 10 to 20 hours if mother has diabetes
    d. timing is dependent on breast stimulation by the baby

25. A mother delivered a preterm baby at 28 weeks gestation. All of the following will be helpful to establish and maintain an adequate milk supply EXCEPT:
    a. begin expressing or pumping within the first 12 hours following birth.
    b. express the breasts fully, for two minutes after the flow of drops ceases.
    c. express or pump every 2 to 4 hours around the clock
    d. pump every 2 hours during the day, and get a good night's sleep at night.

26. Which is the MOST EFFECTIVE strategy for increasing milk supply?
    a. Take fenugreek tea or capsules.
    b. Drink more fluids.
    c. Eat more food.
    d. Hand-express after feeds.

27. A mother asks when she can start giving her baby bovine-based formula so she can go out to a movie. Based on your knowledge of gut closure, your BEST answer is:
    a. after the baby is 6 months old.
    b. after she breastfeeds the baby.
    c. any time, as long as a bottle is not used as the device.
    d. after 1 year of age.

28. When a baby is properly latched-on, where is the tip of the mother's nipple placed in the baby's mouth?
    a. just behind the upper gum ridge
    b. at the center of the hard palate
    c. at the juncture of the hard and soft palates
    d. at the center of the soft palate

29. Which breast structure contains muscle fibers?
    a. lactiferous sinuses
    b. nipple-areola complex
    c. Montgomery tubercles
    d. lobules

30. Which fetal presenting position is the LEAST LIKELY to affect a baby's ability to breastfeed?
    a. left occiput anterior (LOA)
    b. right occiput posterior (ROP)
    c. left mentum anterior (LMA)
    d. right sacrum posterior (RSP)

31. Accessory nipple or breast tissue may be found in any of the following locations EXCEPT:
    a. axilla.
    b. inguinal region.
    c. near the umbillicus.
    d. outer thigh.

32. A mother calls you, frustrated because her three week old baby's preference for nursing at the right breast is so strong that she is unable to get him to nurse on her left side. What is the LEAST likely explanation for this baby's nursing behavior?
    a. There is a subtle positioning difference in the mother's hold on her left side.
    b. The baby has a cephalhematoma on his right side.
    c. The mother has an undetected breast cancer in her left breast.
    d. The baby's right clavicle is fractured.

33. What is the function of the infant's epiglottis during swallowing?
    a. prevents milk from entering the trachea
    b. prevents air from entering the esophagus
    c. propels the bolus of milk to the back of the mouth
    d. traps the bolus of milk, triggering a swallow

34. What is PRIMARILY responsible for the increase in breast size (volume) during pregnancy?
    a. increase in fatty stores in the breast
    b. development of the duct system
    c. growth of secretory epithelial cells
    d. growing uterus triggers ribcage expansion

35. Which structures support the breast on the chest wall?
    a. Bandl's fibers
    b. Cooper's ligaments
    c. mammary ligaments
    d. myoepithelial tissue

36. Lymph drainage from the lactating breast flows to all of the following nodes EXCEPT:
    a. axillary nodes.
    b. intermammary nodes.
    c. subclavicular nodes.
    d. mesenteric nodes.

37. About an hour after collection, bacterial counts in freshly expressed human milk are lower than immediately after collection. The MOST LIKELY explanation for this is:
    a. the cooler temperature in the container is unsuitable for growth of bacteria.
    b. macrophages in milk are actively phagocytic.
    c. gangliosides in milk disrupt the cell walls of bacteria.
    d. bifidus factor starves the bacteria of nutrients.

38. Which of the following is NOT an effect of mother's milk on the child's immune system?
    a. It stimulates baby to begin making his own SigA and other antibodies.
    b. Baby has a better response to immunizations.
    c. It provides passive immunity between placentally acquired immunity and autonomous immune protection.
    d. Baby is protected less because he relies on mother's immune protection during breastfeeding.

39. Women who do not breastfeed their babies are at higher risk for all of the following conditions related to reproduction EXCEPT:
    a. postpartum hemorrhage.
    b. delayed return to prepregnancy weight.
    c. menstrual irregularities and pain.
    d. closely spaced pregnancies.

40. Which of the following statements about the protective aspects of breastfeeding is TRUE?
    a. effective as long as baby is directly breastfeeding
    b. the same whether child is directly breastfed or given breastmilk in a bottle
    c. dose-related for the baby, extending well past the time of direct breastfeeding
    d. available only to the baby, not the mother

41. Which of the following diseases are LEAST LIKELY to be related to artificial feeding?
    a. ulcerative colitis
    b. osteoarthritis
    c. eczema
    d. respiratory infections

42. A mother contracts rubella while breastfeeding her 2-month-old baby. Which of the following actions is MOST appropriate?
    a. Mother should continue breastfeeding.
    b. Mother should immediately stop breastfeeding.
    c. Baby should be isolated from mother.
    d. Mother and baby should immediately receive rubella vaccine.

43. All of these statements accurately describe the protective role of breastfeeding EXCEPT:
    a. the interaction of antiinflammatory and antiinfective factors is more than the sum of its parts.
    b. the unique components of milk protect the mammary gland and the recipient infant from many diseases.
    c. once lactation and breastfeeding cease, the mother and infant are just as vulnerable to disease as anyone else.
    d. protections associated with breastfeeding extend past the time of direct breastfeeding.

44. The risk of which of the following maternal reproductive cancers is NOT reduced by breastfeeding?
    a. cervical cancer
    b. premenopausal breast cancer
    c. ovarian cancer
    d. endometrial cancer

45. A breastfed baby's risk of food allergies is:
    a. decreased, because few food allergens pass through mother's milk.
    b. decreased, because mother's milk makes passage of allergenic proteins through baby's gut less likely.
    c. increased, because allergens pass readily through mother's milk.
    d. increased, because mother's milk increases the permeability of the baby's gut.

46. A breastfeeding mother sustained a broken leg in an automobile injury. Which of the following actions is MOST supportive of breastfeeding after acute care is finished?
    a. Provide her with a hospital-grade electric breastpump.
    b. Encourage family to bring her baby to her for feeding.
    c. Collaborate in selecting pain-relief medications compatible with breastfeeding.
    d. Help the family select an infant formula to use during her hospitalization.

47. Which fetal structure may remain open or be reopened by excessive infant crying?
    a. ductus venosus
    b. ductus arteriosus
    c. foramen ovale
    d. portal sinus

48. Lactoferrin in human milk has all of the following functions EXCEPT:
    a. nutrition.
    b. nerve myelinization.
    c. iron transport.
    d. antiinflammatory agent.

49. Researchers have found that inguinal hernia and some other disorders of the urogenital tract are less common in breastfed babies. Which of the following components has the MOST SIGNIFICANT role in tissue maturation of the infant?
    a. epidermal growth factor
    b. nerve growth factor
    c. secretory IgA
    d. lactoferrin

50. Secretory IgA in mother's milk has all of the following functions EXCEPT:
    a. bind of microbes in baby's gut.
    b. active destruction of bacteria.
    c. antiinflammatory action.
    d. stimulate infant's immune system.

51. Manufacturers of artificial feeding products have attempted to increase the protective properties in their products by adding which of the following nonprotein nitrogen compounds found in human milk?
    a. polyamines
    b. nucleic acids
    c. nucleotides
    d. creatinine

52. The species specificity of human milk is characterized by all of the following EXCEPT:
    a. milk components match 50% of the baby's genetic material.
    b. milk is 75% bioavailable to the infant.
    c. the 200+ identified components have nutritive and immune functions.
    d. milk components meet all the physiological needs of the infant.

53. Which of the following statements BEST describes fetal nutrition?
    a. The umbilical cord delivers nutrients directly to the fetal gut.
    b. The fetus swallows and digests amniotic fluid.
    c. The fetus absorbs nutrients from the amniotic fluid through his skin.
    d. The fetus has no digestive enzymes of his own until after 40 weeks.

54. Most of the antiinfectious properties in human milk perform all of the following EXCEPT:
    a. decrease over the duration of lactation
    b. remain stable over the duration of lactation
    c. are stable to heating or freezing
    d. interact in inhibiting or killing pathogens

55. A mother wants to know how soon she will return to her prepregnant weight after her baby is born. Your responses should include all of the following EXCEPT:
    a. most breastfeeding mothers lose 1 to 2 lbs a week.
    b. making milk uses 1000 calories a day from your diet.
    c. gradual weight loss preserves your health and energy.
    d. do not restrict your calorie intake under 1800 calories a day.

56. You are helping a woman who has a documented allergy to dairy products (cow's milk). Which of the following foods would NOT provide the nutrients lacking in her diet?
    a. rice and potatoes
    b. split peas and lentils
    c. kale and cabbage
    d. corn tortillas soaked in lime

57. Which of the following activities is NOT prohibited by the World Health Organization's International Code of Marketing of Breast-Milk Substitutes?
    a. "gift packs" containing samples and coupons for formula given to new mothers at hospital discharge
    b. detailed information on product composition provided to health workers
    c. advertisements for toddler formula on local television stations
    d. picture of a happy baby on the label of infant formula containers

58. Preterm milk differs from milk of mothers who give birth at term in which of the following ways?
    a. Preterm milk is higher in protein.
    b. Preterm milk is higher in lactose.
    c. Preterm milk is higher in phosphorous.
    d. Preterm milk is higher in iron.

59. Fresh human milk can be instilled in the eye to treat infections. Components in milk that are beneficial for this use include all of the following EXCEPT:
    a. lactose.
    b. fatty acids.
    c. lysozyme.
    d. mucins.

60. A mother is uncertain about providing her own milk for her preterm baby and has been told that her milk helps nerve development. Which sensory system is MOST compromised by the absence of human milk?
    a. olfactory
    b. auditory
    c. taste
    d. visual

61. All of the following components are found in the whey portion of milk EXCEPT:
    a. secretory IgA.
    b. lactoferrin.
    c. docosahexaenoic acid. *fatty acid*
    d. bifidus factor.

62. A pregnant woman follows a vegan diet and intends to breastfeed. You should advise her that:
    a. her milk supply may be compromised by her diet.
    b. she should take a vitamin B12 supplement.
    c. her baby will need a multivitamin supplement.
    d. she will have to change her diet if she wants to breastfeed.

63. Medical uses for donor human milk include all of the following conditions EXCEPT:
    a. post-surgical nutrition.
    b. skin treatment of burns.
    c. solid organ transplants.
    d. allergies and feeding intolerance.

64. A baby born very prematurely (weight 1500 grams or less) is ready to breastfeed when he:
    a. has successfully taken breast milk by bottle.
    b. has first fed by spoon or cup.
    c. is showing sucking movements.
    d. is able to mouth on a pacifier.

65. Additional body contact, such as when the mother uses a soft tie-on type of carrier, is MOST LIKELY to have which of the following effects?
    a. decreased total crying
    b. increased dependency
    c. delayed walking
    d. more night waking

66. A preterm infant of 1361 g (3.0 lbs) has stable cardiac and respiratory systems. All of the following are appropriate EXCEPT:
    a. Begin breastfeeding without equipment or devices.
    b. Breastfeed with nasogastric tube in place.
    c. Cup-feed and allow the baby to suck at an empty breast for comfort.
    d. Bottle-feed with human milk before breastfeeding.

67. Brenda had breast reduction surgery when she was a teenager. Now that she has a new baby, she may need:
    a. a breast pump to relieve engorgement.
    b. a nipple shield to enhance nipple stimulation.
    c. a feeding tube system because of lactation insufficiency.
    d. breast shells to enhance nipple eversion.

68. A mother contacts you for help weaning her baby because she's going back to work in 4 weeks and has no place to express and store her milk. Your responses should include all of the following EXCEPT:
    a. discussion of milk expression techniques and/or equipment.
    b. information on storing milk at room temperature.
    c. encouragement to wean completely.
    d. support for partial breastfeeding during her off-work hours.

69. A 38-week neonate with a birth weight of 3573 g (7 lbs, 12 oz) is referred to you with a discharge weight of 3171 g (6 lbs, 12 oz) at 72 hours post delivery. The FIRST thing you should do is:
    a. weigh the infant to see if the hospital's scale was correct.
    b. tell the mother that the weight loss is within normal range.
    c. take a thorough history of the dyad's breastfeeding practices.
    d. suggest she discuss any interventions with her baby's doctor.

70. You are working with a baby who has a unilateral cleft of the hard palate. The LEAST desirable intervention to suggest is:
    a. instruct the mother on proper attachment, showing her how to fill up the cleft with her breast.
    b. have her supplement with a bottle of artificial baby milk if the baby has difficulty maintaining proper suction at breast.
    c. instruct the mother on proper breast pumping frequency and technique to support her milk supply.
    d. have her feed the baby in upright positions to avoid nasopharyngeal reflux.

71. Freezing human milk destroys which of the following components?
    a. lactoferrin
    b. macrophages
    c. lysozyme
    d. secretory IgA

72. Prematures have the most difficulty digesting which essential nutrient?
    a. carbohydrate
    b. protein
    c. fats
    d. minerals

73. A research article reports that giving a baby one bottle of formula daily between the second and sixth weeks postpartum had no effect on breastfeeding outcomes at 6 weeks. All of the following aspects of the study are flaws that could bring the conclusions into question EXCEPT:
    a. during the protocol period, the planned bottle group gave an average of 5 to 9 bottles per week compared with the total breastfeeding groups' average of less than 2 bottles per week.
    b. in both groups, babies received bottles (a mean of 2 bottles) in the first week postpartum.
    c. no in-person, skilled follow-up care was provided to either group of mothers and babies.
    d. the content of the bottles used (whether formula or mother's own milk) was not consistently documented.

74. An effective, appropriate pamphlet promoting breastfeeding might contain all of the following features EXCEPT:
    a. accurate picture of a baby breastfeeding.
    b. comparison of breastfeeding with artificial feeding.
    c. information about making enough milk.
    d. local sources of breastfeeding help.

75. Which term refers to the middle score in a range of scores?
    a. mean
    b. median
    c. mode
    d. meridian

76. A research study concludes that an event happened purely by chance. Which probability value is MOST LIKELY to show an effect by chance?
    a. $p = 1.0$
    b. $p = 0.10$
    c. $p = 0.01$
    d. $p = 0.001$

77. Which of the following citations is a PRIMARY reference or source?
    a. Anderson GC. Current knowledge about skin-to-skin (Kangaroo) care for preterm infants: review of the literature. *J Perinatol.* 1991; XI: 216-226.
    b. Als H, Lester BM, Tronick E, Brazelton TB. Manual for the assessment of preterm infants' behavior (AFPB). In Fitzgerald JE, Lester BM, Jogman MW, eds. *Theory and Research in Behavioral Pediatrics.* vol 1. New York: Plenum; 1982: 64-133.
    c. Ludington-Hoe SM, Golant SK. *Kangaroo Care: the Best You Can Do to Help Your Preterm Infant.* New York: Bantam Books; 1993.
    d. Ludington-Hoe SM, Hadeed AJ, Anderson GC. Physiologic responses to skin-to-skin contact in hospitalized premature infants. *J Perinatol.* 1991:11(1):19-24

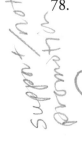

78. Which of the following is NOT an example of breastfeeding promotion?
    a. assisting in developing legislation to protect breastfeeding in public
    b. opening a private lactation practice
    c. presenting a lecture on breastfeeding to a civic organization
    d. wearing breastfeeding buttons, jewelry, or t-shirts in social situations

79. Health care professionals can BEST learn about breastfeeding from all of the following EXCEPT:
    a. conferences sponsored by breastfeeding mother-support organizations or lactation consultant professional associations.
    b. college courses in lactation management
    c. short courses and distance learning programs run by lactation education organizations.
    d. inservice programs presented by scientists employed by formula companies.

80. The existing policy on the maternity unit at your hospital is to supplement all breastfeeding babies with 1 oz (30 ml) glucose water by bottle after every breastfeed. The strategy that is LEAST likely to be effective in changing this policy is to:
    a. include pediatricians, nursing staff, and neonatalogists on the policy planning committee.
    b. distribute copies of research articles from peer-reviewed journals on the subject.
    c. plan a series of inservices for all affected staff to carefully educate them on the risks and benefits of supplementing breastfeeding babies.
    d. develop the new policy with a small core group, then tell the staff that they must follow the new policy.

81. Which of the following provisions is NOT part of the International Labor Organization's Maternity Protection Convention?
    a. 12 weeks maternity leave
    b. two half-hour nursing breaks
    c. on-site child care
    d. job security after maternity leave

82. The WHO/UNICEF Ten Steps to Successful Breastfeeding (Baby Friendly Hospital Initiative) prohibits the use of all of the following devices EXCEPT:
    a. artificial teats (nipples).
    b. pacifiers (dummies, soothers).
    c. breast pumps.
    d. feeding bottles.

83. Which of the following practices is an appropriate precaution to take in the hospital labor and delivery (birthing) unit?
    a. Make sure the baby can take formula by bottle before attempting to breastfeed.
    b. Read the hospital policies to the mother before she is admitted in labor.
    c. Deep suction the baby before feeding with oral fluids, including breastmilk or colostrum.
    d. Give the baby only mother's own milk or colostrum unless medically indicated.

84. A mother of a fussy, gassy baby has been drinking 10 glasses of cow's milk per day on her doctor's recommendation. Your FIRST action would be:
    a. encourage her to follow her doctor's dietary advice.
    b. take a thorough history, including allergy and food sensitivity in the family.
    c. tell her that 6 to 8 glasses of any liquid is adequate during lactation.
    d. tell her that consumption of dairy products is not related to her baby's symptoms.

85. You are about to assess a breastfeeding mother and her baby. What should you do FIRST?
    a. obtain written consent from the mother
    b. weigh the baby
    c. examine the mother's breasts
    d. wash your hands

86. A lactation consultant (LC) operates a private breastpump rental depot from her home. She is also a staff nurse in a hospital maternity unit. When a mother leaves the hospital without her baby, the LC tells the mother about her own rental depot but not others in the community. This behavior is:
    a. legal and ethical.
    b. illegal and unethical.
    c. a conflict of interest.
    d. a valuable service to patients.

87. You are a private practice lactation consultant and you have just received word that a couple to whom you provided LC services is suing you for malpractice. The FIRST thing you should do is:
    a. call an attorney.
    b. contact your professional malpractice insurance agent.
    c. talk to the couple to find out why they are upset.
    d. speak to the couple's physician.

88. A mother of 10-week-old twins calls. She says that all she does all day is feed babies and she can't take it anymore. She asks how she can introduce some artificial baby milk or infant cereal without weaning her babies from the breast. The FIRST thing you should do is:
    a. suggest she feed her infants simultaneously in order to save time.
    b. tell her that offering other foods will decrease milk production.
    c. ask if she has any help with household chores.
    d. actively listen, and praise her for breastfeeding two babies.

89. Which aspect of maternal-infant bonding with mothers of multiple infants is most likely to occur FIRST?
    a. mother bonds with the unit
    b. mother bonds with the firstborn
    c. mother bonds with the lastborn
    d. mother has delayed bonding with all

90. Employers with breastfeeding support programs for employees are likely to experience all of the following EXCEPT:
    a. reduced employee absenteeism.
    b. reduced employee productivity.
    c. increased retention of employees.
    d. increased employee morale.

91. You have been collaborating with a physician regarding a breastfeeding mother who experienced a psychotic episode. The question is whether or not she should continue to breastfeed during drug treatment. The drug prescribed is considered compatible with breastfeeding. Your BEST response is:
    a. Breastfeeding may be healing for her under carefully controlled conditions.
    b. Breastfeeding is contraindicated for mothers with mental illnesses.
    c. Her baby is in great danger and should be kept away from her at all costs.
    d. The hormones of breastfeeding will exacerbate her illness.

92. A mother asks for your help with weaning her toddler. Your responses should include all of the following EXCEPT:
    a. For both you and him, it is best to wean gradually.
    b. Put some bitter substance on your nipples to discourage him.
    c. Let's look for other ways to meet his needs for closeness.
    d. Be aware that your fertility will likely return in a few weeks.

93. A mother tells you "Breastfeeding has been so wonderful! Now I want to talk to every pregnant woman and tell her to breastfeed!" This statement is an example of:
    a. overenthusiasm.
    b. empowerment.
    c. delusion of grandeur.
    d. self-actualization.

94. A mother is concerned that her baby has suddenly lost interest in breastfeeding. Your BEST response is:
     a. do nothing. Breastfeeding mothers are usually overprotective.
     b. reassure her that babies appetite may change abruptly.
     c. carefully investigate the situation.
     d. instruct her how to give her milk in a bottle.

95. A mother calls in a panic on day 3. She has been crying all morning, her breasts hurt, and her baby is having a hard time feeding. Your FIRST response to her should be:
     a. How many times did your baby stool today?
     b. Things sure are overwhelming for you today!
     c. Have you been pumping your breasts?
     d. You'll be fine—lots of mothers have problems on day 3.

96. Twenty-four hour rooming-in from birth has been shown to have all the following effects EXCEPT:
     a. increased maternal-infant bonding (attachment).
     b. increased duration of breastfeeding.
     c. decreased abandonment or neglect of infant.
     d. decreased interaction between grandparents and baby.

97. A mother of a 10-week-old adopted baby consults you inquiring about induced lactation. The FIRST thing you would tell her is:
     a. adoptive breastfeeding is possible.
     b. the baby is the deciding factor.
     c. how to provide supplementary feeds.
     d. she won't have a full milk supply.

98. Early feeding cues include all of the following EXCEPT:
     a. crying.
     b. hand-to-face or hand-to-mouth.
     c. grope or mouthing motions.
     d. moving into feeding position.

99. Compared with the NCHS growth charts used for many years, which statement BEST describe the growth of exclusively breastfed babies in the first 6 months?
     a. Breastfed babies gain more weight.
     b. Breastfed babies are longer in length.
     c. There is no difference in weight gain.
     d. Breastfed babies are leaner per height.

100. A 3-week old, exclusively breastfed baby nurses every 1.5 to 2 hours in the late afternoon and evenings. She is gaining over 1 oz per day with 5 to 6 profuse, yellow stools and 8+ wet diapers per day. The MOST LIKELY explanation for this frequent nursing pattern is :
    a. normal behavior for this age.
    b. low milk supply.
    c. baby is becoming too dependent.
    d. baby is ready for solid foods.

101. The mother of a 4-month-old exclusively breastfed baby wonders when her baby will sleep through the night without waking to feed. Your BEST response is:
    a. by the time he is 6 months old.
    b. when he has doubled his birthweight.
    c. when you stop nursing him as soon as he cries.
    d. when he is physiologically ready.

102. All of the following statements about nursing strikes are true EXCEPT:
    a. may occur between 7 and 9 months of age.
    b. may coincide with infant illness.
    c. with careful attention, baby will usually go back to breast.
    d. the baby is indicating readiness to wean.

103. The MOST LIKELY cause of inadequate milk supply is:
    a. impaired let-down reflex.
    b. restricted maternal fluid intake.
    c. inadequate or infrequent milk removal.
    d. inadequate maternal diet.

104. Breastfeeding a child for more than 2 years:
    a. provides no immune protection to the child.
    b. provides health benefits to mother and child.
    c. prolongs the child's dependency on mother.
    d. increases incidence of tooth decay.

105. The mother of a 5-month-old breastfeeding baby is MOST LIKELY to observe that the baby:
    a. plays with the mother's other nipple while breastfeeding.
    b. closes her eyes during breastfeeding.
    c. is easily distracted while nursing.
    d. does not awaken to breastfeed at night.

106. Which of the following statements BEST describes the Babinski reflex?
     a. grasp object when palm is stimulated
     b. turn mouth toward source of stimulation
     c. bear partial weight of body while standing on flat surface
     d. flare toes when sole of foot is stimulated

107. A pregnant woman and her husband both have many allergies. She asks whether there is anything she can do to reduce her child's risks of allergic disease. Your responses should include all of the following EXCEPT:
     a. avoid common allergens such as cow's milk during your pregnancy.
     b. exclusively breastfeed for at least 6 months.
     c. continue breastfeeding to at least 24 months or longer if your child is willing.
     d. take steroid medications to strengthen your immune system.

108. A baby born at 32 weeks gestation was growing normally for 2 weeks, and then his growth began slowing. The LEAST LIKELY cause of this sudden slow weight gain is:
     a. exclusive use of human milk.
     b. respiratory infection.
     c. necrotizing enterocolitis.
     d. cardiac anomaly.

109. How long does it take the infant gut to recover its normal flora after ONE bottle of artificial baby milk?
     a. 2 feedings
     b. 2 days
     c. 2 weeks
     d. 2 months

110. When a mother is giving birth to twins, the LEAST LIKELY reason that the second baby might have a problem initiating breastfeeding is:
     a. higher likelihood of prolapsed cord.
     b. malpresentation causing birth injury.
     c. mother is busy with the first-born twin.
     d. the second baby is usually the smaller of the two.

111. The implications of breastfeeding the infant of a treatment-controlled mother with hyperthyroidism are:
    a. the baby should not be breastfed.
    b. the baby may be breastfed, but should be monitored for hyperthyroidism.
    c. the baby may breastfeed normally.
    d. the baby will need thyroid medication.

112. Which infant disease is incompatible with breastfeeding?
    a. hypythyroidism
    b. Down syndrome
    c. phenylketonuria
    d. galactosemia

113. A baby gained 19 ounces in the past 5 days but is fussy and gassy much of the day. His mother feeds him on both breasts at each feed. Your BEST suggestion to her is:
    a. Cut down your own fluid intake, because you have too much milk.
    b. Let him finish nursing on the first breast before you offer the other one.
    c. Stop drinking cow's milk for the next two weeks.
    d. Try giving him some lactose-free supplement three times a day.

114. The management of mother-baby couples addressed in the WHO/UNICEF Baby Friendly Hospital Initiative (Ten Steps to Successful Breastfeeding) applies to:
    a. all babies, no matter how fed.
    b. all artificially fed babies.
    c. all breastfed babies.
    d. breastfed babies who room-in.

115. Breastfeeding protects the infant from allergy by all of the following methods EXCEPT:
    a. limiting the baby's exposure to nonhuman proteins.
    b. slowing or preventing the absorption of allergens through the baby's gut.
    c. protecting the baby's gut from inflammation, which weakens the mucosal barrier.
    d. providing white cells in milk which attack the allergens directly.

116. For optimal breastfeeding, all of the following structures need to be positioned inside the infant's mouth EXCEPT:
    a. nipple epithelium.
    b. areola.
    c. milk duct outlets.
    d. alveoli.

117. The standard temperature and time for Holder pasteurization used in human milk banks is:
    a. 56 degrees Celsius for 20 minutes.
    b. 61.4 degrees Celsius 25 minutes.
    c. 62.5 degrees Celsius for 30 minutes.
    d. 58.6 degrees Celsius for 30 minutes.

118. Exclusive breastfeeding means that:
    a. mother's milk is transferred directly from her breast to her infant's mouth.
    b. baby receives only his mother's milk, either directly or from devices when mother is away.
    c. baby receives less than 2 oz (60 ml) of other fluids per day.
    d. baby receives no formula or solid foods.

119. What is the average percentage of a drug administered to a lactating woman that actually gets to the breastfeeding baby?
    a. 0.01%
    b. 0.1%
    c. 1.0%
    d. 10%

120. Breastfeeding is usually contraindicated when the mother is taking which category of drug?
    a. antimicrobial
    b. antihypertensive
    c. antineoplastic
    d. antidepressant

121. Local perineal injection of an anesthetic drug prior to performing an episiotomy may have all the following consequences EXCEPT:
    a. mother's discomfort sitting up to feed.
    b. infant bradycardia due to the medication used.
    c. increased risk of perineal infection.
    d. tissue damage from the procedure.

122. A lactating mother noticed two raised bumps on her areola that drip milk when her baby is nursing on the other breast. These bumps are MOST LIKELY:
    a. Montgomery glands
    b. milk duct pores
    c. warts
    d. insect bites

123. When you see this condition in a breastfeeding infant, all of the following recommendations are appropriate EXCEPT:
    a. Begin simultaneous treatment of the baby and mother's breast.
    b. Unless the mother has signs of infection, treat only the baby's mouth with an antifungal medication.
    c. Check mother's nipples for signs or symptoms of infection.
    d. Assume that mother's nipples, all infant sucking objects, and possibly other infant areas are infected until proved otherwise.

124. You have just observed this mother feeding her baby. She describes nipple pain all throughout the feed. At the next feed, you would suggest all of the following EXCEPT:
    a. bring the baby onto the breast more deeply.
    b. wait till the baby's mouth is very widely open before latching.
    c. everything looks good—do what you've been doing all along.
    d. make sure the baby's lip is turned outward (flanged).

125. This full-term baby is 36 hours old. The MOST LIKELY condition requiring this treatment is:
    a. breastmilk jaundice.
    b. ABO incompatibility.
    c. exclusive breastfeeding.
    d. hypoglycemia.

126. Which statement is LEAST LIKELY to be true concerning this mother's breast and nipple?
    a. The nipple is flat.
    b. The nipple/areolar complex has poor elasticity.
    c. The nipple tip is very soft and pliable.
    d. The nipple inverts between feeds.

127. The baby's mother complains of sore nipples. Of the following, which is the FIRST question you should ask?
    a. May I watch you breastfeed right now?
    b. Did you prepare your nipples during pregnancy?
    c. Are you feeling a stinging, itching sensation?
    d. How long do you intend to breastfeed?

128. This activity is appropriate or necessary during which of the following maternal conditions?
    a. Chickenpox
    b. Infectious mastitis
    c. Breast abscess near the nipple
    d. Toxoplasmosis

129. This picture was taken immediately after a baby ended a feeding. Which statement MOST LIKELY describes the preceeding feed?
    a. comfortable, with good milk transfer
    b. comfortable, but with poor milk transfer
    c. painful, but with good milk transfer
    d. painful, with poor milk transfer

130. Documentation of this woman's breasts might include all of the following EXCEPT:
    a. Breasts are asymmetric with a pinkish nipple/areola complex.
    b. Right breast is very small; left breast is moderate size and saggy.
    c. Both breasts have scant palpable glandular tissue.
    d. Right breast has insufficient glandular tissue for lactation.

131. What is the MOST LIKELY explanation for the condition pictured?
    a. milk residue after pumping
    b. nipple candidiasis
    c. herpes lesions
    d. lanolin

132. What is the MOST LIKELY condition pictured?
    a. candida infection at the base of the nipple
    b. large, fibrous nipple
    c. nipple edema from excessive pumping
    d. scars from breast reduction surgery

133. What is the MOST LIKELY cause of the dark marks on this mother's areola?
    a. herpes lesions
    b. tooth marks from toddler's biting
    c. bruise (ecchymosis) from baby's off-center latch
    d. improper use of breast pump

134. On day 6 (as pictured), this mother says she is enjoying breastfeed-
      ing. Your FIRST response should be:
      a. Your baby looks a bit jaundiced—has he seen the doctor?
      b. How many times has your baby nursed in the past 24 hours?
      c. How many wet diapers have you changed so far today?
      d. Wonderful! You were ambivalent, and now you look so confi-
          dent. How are things going?

135. Which of the following is MOST associated with this sleep position?
      a. increased time in deep sleep
      b. less risk of sudden infant death syndrome
      c. less chance of aspiration of milk
      d. decreased number of awakenings at night

136. This mother is worried about her full-term baby's skin color. Your
      BEST recommendation is:
      a. have the baby's bilirubin checked by the pediatrician.
      b. adjust her positioning and encourage breastfeeding every 1 to 3
          hours.
      c. have her begin supplementing feeds with expressed breastmilk.
      d. have her give the baby water between breastfeeds.

137. This child's mother wonders why her child recently became ill with a
      respiratory illness. Your BEST response is:
      a. the immune factors in human milk decrease after 6 months.
      b. as his mobility increases, he is exposed to more pathogens.
      c. teething lowers his resistance to infection.
      d. placentally acquired immunity is wearing off.

138. Which situation is LEAST LIKELY to cause the condition shown?
      a. baby has a short, tight frenulum
      b. shallow latch
      c. flat, inelastic nipple tissue
      d. biting during nursing

139. This mother is concerned about the condition on her breast, which
      suddenly appeared when her baby was 4 months old. You should
      take all of the following actions EXCEPT:
      a. visually examine the baby's mouth and throat.
      b. take a thorough history of the mother and baby.
      c. give her a topical steroid cream to reduce inflammation.
      d. recommend that she get a medical evaluation.

140. This mother-infant dyad needs to be carefully assessed for:
    a. duration of feeds.
    b. thrush.
    c. nipple shield use.
    d. latch-on technique.

141. The behavior exhibited by this baby often occurs about 2 hours after the last breastfeed. What is your BEST recommendation to the mother?
    a. Offer her a pacifier to satisfy her need to suck.
    b. Breastfeed her again, now.
    c. Let her cry a bit so her feedings get spaced out.
    d. Give her some water to tide her over until the next feed.

142. According to the Baby-Friendly Hospital Initiative, this event should take place no more than:
    a. 10 minutes after birth.
    b. 1 hour after birth.
    c. 6 hours after birth.
    d. 12 hours after birth.

143. What is the FIRST suggestion you would give this mother?
    a. Use a nipple shield during feeds.
    b. Have your baby's suck evaluated immediately.
    c. Keep up the good work—everything looks great.
    d. Bring your baby deeper onto your breast.

144. This baby has been at breast about 25 minutes. What is your BEST recommendation to this mother?
    a. Insert your finger to break the suction, then remove him.
    b. Pull his buttocks in closer to you for a better latch.
    c. Watch his sucking slow down as he prepares to self-detach.
    d. Tickle his feet to wake him so he can finish the feed.

145. This mother is 4 days postbirth. What is the MOST LIKELY cause of the condition pictured?
    a. plugged milk duct
    b. infected sweat gland in axilla
    c. mastitis in the tail of Spence
    d. milk stasis in accessory breast tissue

146. This practice has all of the following results on the infant's physiology EXCEPT:
    a. higher infant metabolism.
    b. reduced infant pain.
    c. stabilized infant temperature.
    d. increased infant oxygen saturation.

147. This breastfeeding mother recently became pregnant again. Her child (pictured) breastfeeds several times a day and once or twice at night. She calls you to find a solution for suddenly sore nipples. Your FIRST comment should be:
    a. You'll need to wean your toddler because continued breastfeeding might cause a miscarriage.
    b. The tenderness is probably because of pregnancy hormones. How much of a problem is this for you?
    c. Is your toddler teething? His saliva may be irritating to your nipples now.
    d. Have you or he recently taken an antibiotic?

148. Which of the following statements BEST describes the exclusively breastfed baby of this age?
    a. will need complementary (solid) food soon
    b. takes about 80% of available milk over the course of a day
    c. needs vitamin D supplements
    d. is at highest risk of SIDS

149. What is the name of the string-like structure under this baby's tongue?
    a. labial frenulum
    b. incisive papilla
    c. lingual frenulum
    d. mucus membrane

150. This baby is 1 day old. In this picture, what are the white things in its mouth?
    a. Epstein's pearls
    b. natal teeth
    c. incisive papilla
    d. sucking blisters

151. Which statement MOST ACCURATELY describes this baby's oral anatomy?
    a. The fat pads are too small.
    b. The philtrim is too broad.
    c. The lips are too thin and tensed.
    d. All visible structures are normal.

152. The pale-colored lumps on this mother's breast are MOST LIKELY:
    a. lipomas.
    b. plugged pores.
    c. Montgomery's tubercles.
    d. warts.

153. The LEAST LIKELY cause of this nipple wound is:
    a. baby was nursing on the nipple tip.
    b. baby is tongue-tied.
    c. no nipple preparation during pregnancy.
    d. use of a pacifier between feeds.

154. During breastfeeding, this baby's mother has noticed loud clicking and smacking. This could be caused by all of the following EXCEPT:
    a. prominent buccal fat pads compromising tongue motion.
    b. oddly shaped tongue tip, causing loss of seal during sucking.
    c. short, tight labial frenulum preventing deep attachment at breast.
    d. tight muscles around the mouth, causing overuse of lips to create seal.

155. What is the MOST LIKELY cause of the condition shown?
    a. bacterial infection
    b. allergic reaction from laundry soap
    c. friction damage from baby's tongue
    d. mother has fair skin

156. This woman says the condition pictured on her inner thigh becomes tender about once a month. It is MOST LIKELY:
    a. skin tag responding to varying estrogen levels.
    b. wart that is sensitive to her clothing.
    c. mole that should be examined by a dermatologist.
    d. accessory nipple with sensitivity paralleling menstrual cycles.

157. What is the MOST LIKELY condition pictured?
    a. abcess in the lower inner quadrant of the left breast
    b. bilateral primary engorgement
    c. large breasts with accessory breast tissue in both axilla
    d. bilateral mastitis extending to the axilla

158. This baby is having difficulty latching on and breastfeeding. The MOST LIKELY reason is:
    a. the baby is crying too hard to latch well.
    b. the lingual frenulum is restricting tongue movement.
    c. the lips are too tense.
    d. the baby's mouth is not open wide enough.

159. This exclusively breastfed baby is gaining well and otherwise healthy. For the condition pictured, your BEST recommendation to the mother is:
    a. Try eliminating dairy from your diet for a week to rule out an allergic response.
    b. Give the baby water between breastfeeds because her urine is too concentrated.
    c. Start supplementing with soy formula because your milk supply is inadequate.
    d. Put her in a crib at night so she learns to sleep longer at a stretch.

160. Which of the following findings is MOST LIKELY to be related to this mother's breastfeeding problem?
    a. Her husband has an oral yeast infection.
    b. The baby recently had strep throat.
    c. Her baby is 7 months old and teething.
    d. The mother has many allergies, including atopic dermatitis.

161. The MOST LIKELY result of this mother's dietary practices would be:
    a. her milk will contain more vitamin A.
    b. her milk supply will increase.
    c. the baby's breath may smell like cantaloupe.
    d. the baby will reject the cantaloupe-flavored milk.

162. The breastfeeding equipment shown in this photograph is MOST LIKELY being used for:
    a. provision of sufficient calories while increasing the milk supply.
    b. training the baby at the breast to suck correctly and effectively.
    c. ensuring adequate caloric intake because this baby is too small to obtain enough nourishment.
    d. aiding this baby to attach correctly to the breast and continue sucking.

163. This baby now refuses to take a bottle from her day care provider. Your BEST recommendation to her mother is that the provider should:
    a. give milk in a cup.
    b. wait until the child is really hungry.
    c. try an orthodontic-shaped teat (nipple).
    d. give the bottle in a dark room.

164. This technique is recommended for all the following conditions EXCEPT:
    a. Down syndrome.
    b. premature baby.
    c. mother with nipple thrush.
    d. giving medication to infant.

165. To comfortably breastfeed, this mother may want to use:
    a. a breastpump to remove excessive milk before feeding.
    b. ice packs to reduce swelling.
    c. a nipple shield to help her baby latch on.
    d. a well-fitting bra to support her large breasts.

166. To properly use this device, the mother should:
    a. cycle the pressure about 40 to 60 times per minute.
    b. hold the pressure steady for up to 5 seconds.
    c. cycle the pressure about 80 to 100 times per minute.
    d. use the pump vacuum to stretch the breast forward.

167. The adult's hand is MOST LIKELY doing which of these procedures?
    a. suck training or reorganization
    b. digital oral exam or assessment
    c. finger-feeding
    d. pacifying a crying/upset baby

168. This baby is having trouble feeding. Which suggestion is MOST LIKELY to improve the situation?
    a. Mother should support her breast with her left hand.
    b. Pull baby's hips and legs in closer to mom's body.
    c. Place a pillow under baby's body.
    d. Change to a horizontal position.

169. This mother complains of severe pain at latch-on and continuing during the entire feed. What is the FIRST thing you would do?
    a. Attempt deeper attachment at breast.
    b. Make sure she breaks the baby's suction at the end of feeds.
    c. Weigh the baby before and after the next two consecutive feeds.
    d. Try nursing lying down instead of sitting up.

170. Which visual element of this baby's latch is MOST LIKELY to indicate a problem?
    a. deep puckering at the nasolabial crease
    b. eyes are closed
    c. chin is driven into the breast
    d. nose is barely touching the breast

171. This baby has difficulty latching on to the breast and cannot sustain a sucking pattern for more than a few minutes. Which of the following suggestions would be LEAST LIKELY to help this baby breast-feed?
    a. Position the baby in a vertical position with his head higher than his shoulders.
    b. Reduce light and sound in the room.
    c. Feed expressed mother's milk with an orthodontic shaped teat (nipple).
    d. Handle the baby gently and slowly as if he has a headache.

172. This mother complains of sudden onset sore nipples. The FIRST action you would take is:
    a. ask whether her baby has teeth.
    b. roll her inward toward you, so her entire front side is facing yours.
    c. pull her legs in closer to you.
    d. ask whether she has taken an antibiotic recently.

173. This mother's baby is 4 months old. The LEAST APPROPRIATE suggestion you would offer this mother is:
    a. See your doctor or a dermatologist for a diagnosis of these rashes.
    b. Have your baby's mouth cultured for possible infectious organisms.
    c. Keep a diary of all the foods you and your baby are eating.
    d. Start using a breastpump and feed the collected milk to the baby by another means.

174. Consequences of using this equipment include all of the following EXCEPT:
    a. release of stress hormones in the baby.
    b. neonatal hypothermia.
    c. facilitates maternal access to infant.
    d. increased crying.

175. To relieve the condition pictured, your BEST recommendation is:
    a. Hand-express for a few minutes before each feed.
    b. Soak your nipples in warm water then gently massage the tip.
    c. Wear breast shells between feeds.
    d. Apply an antifungal preparation after each feed.

176.   Which action or statement would be MOST HELPFUL to this mother?
   a.   Try to get all of your areola into the baby's mouth.
   b.   Remove your bra so the baby can get a deep latch.
   c.   Support your breast from underneath, between your thumb and first finger.
   d.   Center your nipple in the baby's mouth and lean forward to help him latch.

177.   This woman is in her third trimester of pregnancy. What is the MOST IMPORTANT action you could take to help her prepare to breastfeed?
   a.   Teach her good positioning and latch-on technique, using a doll as a model.
   b.   Provide her with breast shells to wear several hours a day.
   c.   Teach her Hoffman's techniques to prepare her nipples.
   d.   Instruct her to rub her nipples with a towel several times a day.

178.   This mother is preparing to feed. The NEXT action she should take is:
   a.   rub the nipple to make it firmer and more projectile.
   b.   move the bottom hand closer to the areola to better support the breast.
   c.   stop pulling back with the top hand.
   d.   bring the baby onto the breast.

179.   What is the FIRST suggestion you would make to help this mother breastfeed more comfortably?
   a.   Place a nipple shield over your nipple until the baby's suck improves.
   b.   Wear a supportive bra 24 hours a day.
   c.   Support your breast with your hand during feeds.
   d.   Use some lanolin on your nipple before feeds.

180.   This baby's mother calls you, worried because for the past 2 days her baby has been nursing much more frequently than previously. The MOST likely reason for the change in nursing pattern is:
   a.   teething.
   b.   illness.
   c.   growth spurt.
   d.   need for supplemental foods.

181. The MOST LIKELY explanation for what this mother is doing is:
    a. doing a pinch test for retraction.
    b. doing nipple rolling technique.
    c. measuring the size of her areola.
    d. hand-expressing her milk.

182. How is the baby pictured responding to this technique?
    a. stressed
    b. shut down
    c. relaxed
    d. agitated

183. The MOST APPROPRIATE advice you can give this mother on feeding patterns is:
    a. Your milk supply is very high, so use only one breast per feed.
    b. Start on the fuller breast for about 10 minutes, then switch to the other.
    c. Let the baby nurse on the first breast until he self-detaches.
    d. Switch sides several times during a feed to make sure both sides get stimulated.

184. This mother brings her baby to a well-child clinic for a routine visit and nurses in the position shown. Your FIRST response should be any of the following EXCEPT:
    a. How is breastfeeding going for you both?
    b. Turn your baby's body to face your body.
    c. Has your baby shown an interest in family foods?
    d. What family planning method are you using or planning to use?

185. According to the Ten Steps to Successful Breastfeeding, this baby should be:
    a. brought to the admission nursery only after 1 hour.
    b. moved to the central nursery only if the mother had a cesarean birth.
    c. given eye phophylaxis when over 2 hours of age.
    d. kept with the mother 24 hours a day.

186. Common breastfeeding behaviors of babies at this age include all of the following EXCEPT:
    a. playing with toes while nursing.
    b. increased sucking need.
    c. handling mother's other breast.
    d. lifting mother's shirt/blouse.

187. This mother has been warned that she is spoiling her baby by using the device in the picture. Which of the following statements about this practice is FALSE?
    a. Continuous body contact helps the baby maintain body temperature.
    b. Carrying in a sling allows the baby easy access to breastfeeding.
    c. Carrying reduces infant crying.
    d. Carrying prolongs dependency of the baby on its mother.

188. At this postdelivery stage, it is MOST LIKELY that:
    a. too many visitors can interfere with feeding.
    b. mother is getting ready to go back to work.
    c. baby can't consume all the milk that mother is making.
    d. baby is sleeping 6 to 8 hours at night.

189. You are caring for this mother and baby. The baby is 4 hours old and has breastfed well shortly after birth. Upon entering this mother's room, the FIRST THING you should do is:
    a. attempt to wake the baby for another feeding.
    b. check the baby's blood glucose by doing a heel stick.
    c. quietly observe the mother and baby but do not intervene.
    d. have the mother put the baby in a crib next to the bed.

190. This mother is uncomfortable in this situation. Your BEST response to her is:
    a. You'll get used to it—many mothers breastfeed in public.
    b. You could always try the ladies' room.
    c. It won't hurt to give the baby a bottle when you're out shopping.
    d. It can be embarrassing the first few times you breastfeed away from home.

191. The kind of care being given to this laboring woman results in all of the following EXCEPT:
    a. reduced involvement by her husband (partner).
    b. longer duration of breast feeding.
    c. lower risk of cesarean birth.
    d. less infant asphyxia.

192. A child of the age shown is MOST LIKELY to be developmentally ready to:
    a. crawl and attempt to stand alone.
    b. wean from the breast.
    c. sleep through the night alone.
    d. separate easily from mother.

193. Which behavior is LEAST LIKELY to occur in the breastfeeding child shown in this picture?
    a. breastfeeding 8 to 12 times per 24 hours
    b. sleeping through the night
    c. separation anxiety
    d. self-feeding of family foods

194. The behavior shown in this picture is LEAST likely to be:
    a. distress at separation from mother.
    b. an indication of pain.
    c. infant's attempt to manipulate mother.
    d. stressful to the baby's physiology.

195. This mother has been told that her baby should no longer feed at night. Your BEST response to her is:
    a. It's time to begin solid foods.
    b. Try and get him to nurse more in the daytime.
    c. Use a pacifier during the night.
    d. This is normal behavior.

196. If her mother moves the dog's water dish out of her sight, this child will:
    a. crawl straight to it.
    b. forget it was there.
    c. become confused.
    d. search for it without knowing where to look.

197. The interaction shown between this woman and baby begins at which age?
    a. 1 day
    b. 1 week
    c. 2 weeks
    d. 1 month

198. Which of the following breastfeeding-related behaviors is this baby MOST LIKELY to exhibit?
    a. gazes up and smiles at mother
    b. hands relax as baby obtains milk
    c. reaches for mother's face
    d. cues to feed by crying

199. This mother is getting irritated with her child's nursing habits. The child is afraid of strangers, cries when left with a caregiver, and wakes several times at night. The MOST LIKELY reason for this behavior pattern is:
     a.   delayed development of autonomy caused by breastfeeding.
     b.   mother clinging to her child and discouraging autonomy.
     c.   common and normal behavior in the second 6 months of life.
     d.   mother's inability to set limits for the child's behavior.

200. Which of the following statements about this practice is FALSE?
     a.   helps the baby maintain body temperature
     b.   allows the baby easy access to breastfeeding
     c.   reduces infant crying
     d.   prolongs dependency on the mother

YOUR SCORE

To self-grade your exam: Compare your answers to the Answer Key. Circle any *wrong* answers.

Total number of questions	200
Your number of *wrong* answers	————
Subtract number of wrong answers from 200	
Total number of correct answers	————
Multiply each correct answer by 0.5	———— x.05

Your Score ————

The passing grade for this exam simulation is 65%.

Congratulations if you passed!

If you did not get a score of 65 or higher, use the answer key to identify your areas of weakness, focus your study efforts in those areas, and retake the examination simulation to check your progress.

GENERAL PURPOSE - NCS® - ANSWER SHEET
SEE IMPORTANT MARKING INSTRUCTIONS ON SIDE 2

SIDE 1

NAME (Last, First, M.I.)

BIRTHDATE — MO. DAY YR.

IDENTIFICATION NUMBER

SPECIAL CODES

120

SIDE 2

GENERAL PURPOSE NCS®

ANSWER SHEET

form no. 4521

A B C D E	A B C D E	A B C D E	A B C D E	A B C D E
101 ① ② ③ ④ ⑤	111 ① ② ③ ④ ⑤	121 ① ② ③ ④ ⑤	131 ① ② ③ ④ ⑤	141 ① ② ③ ④ ⑤
102 ① ② ③ ④ ⑤	112 ① ② ③ ④ ⑤	122 ① ② ③ ④ ⑤	132 ① ② ③ ④ ⑤	142 ① ② ③ ④ ⑤
103 ① ② ③ ④ ⑤	113 ① ② ③ ④ ⑤	123 ① ② ③ ④ ⑤	133 ① ② ③ ④ ⑤	143 ① ② ③ ④ ⑤
104 ① ② ③ ④ ⑤	114 ① ② ③ ④ ⑤	124 ① ② ③ ④ ⑤	134 ① ② ③ ④ ⑤	144 ① ② ③ ④ ⑤
105 ① ② ③ ④ ⑤	115 ① ② ③ ④ ⑤	125 ① ② ③ ④ ⑤	135 ① ② ③ ④ ⑤	145 ① ② ③ ④ ⑤
106 ① ② ③ ④ ⑤	116 ① ② ③ ④ ⑤	126 ① ② ③ ④ ⑤	136 ① ② ③ ④ ⑤	146 ① ② ③ ④ ⑤
107 ① ② ③ ④ ⑤	117 ① ② ③ ④ ⑤	127 ① ② ③ ④ ⑤	137 ① ② ③ ④ ⑤	147 ① ② ③ ④ ⑤
108 ① ② ③ ④ ⑤	118 ① ② ③ ④ ⑤	128 ① ② ③ ④ ⑤	138 ① ② ③ ④ ⑤	148 ① ② ③ ④ ⑤
109 ① ② ③ ④ ⑤	119 ① ② ③ ④ ⑤	129 ① ② ③ ④ ⑤	139 ① ② ③ ④ ⑤	149 ① ② ③ ④ ⑤
110 ① ② ③ ④ ⑤	120 ① ② ③ ④ ⑤	130 ① ② ③ ④ ⑤	140 ① ② ③ ④ ⑤	150 ① ② ③ ④ ⑤
151 ① ② ③ ④ ⑤	161 ① ② ③ ④ ⑤	171 ① ② ③ ④ ⑤	181 ① ② ③ ④ ⑤	191 ① ② ③ ④ ⑤
152 ① ② ③ ④ ⑤	162 ① ② ③ ④ ⑤	172 ① ② ③ ④ ⑤	182 ① ② ③ ④ ⑤	192 ① ② ③ ④ ⑤
153 ① ② ③ ④ ⑤	163 ① ② ③ ④ ⑤	173 ① ② ③ ④ ⑤	183 ① ② ③ ④ ⑤	193 ① ② ③ ④ ⑤
154 ① ② ③ ④ ⑤	164 ① ② ③ ④ ⑤	174 ① ② ③ ④ ⑤	184 ① ② ③ ④ ⑤	194 ① ② ③ ④ ⑤
155 ① ② ③ ④ ⑤	165 ① ② ③ ④ ⑤	175 ① ② ③ ④ ⑤	185 ① ② ③ ④ ⑤	195 ① ② ③ ④ ⑤
156 ① ② ③ ④ ⑤	166 ① ② ③ ④ ⑤	176 ① ② ③ ④ ⑤	186 ① ② ③ ④ ⑤	196 ① ② ③ ④ ⑤
157 ① ② ③ ④ ⑤	167 ① ② ③ ④ ⑤	177 ① ② ③ ④ ⑤	187 ① ② ③ ④ ⑤	197 ① ② ③ ④ ⑤
158 ① ② ③ ④ ⑤	168 ① ② ③ ④ ⑤	178 ① ② ③ ④ ⑤	188 ① ② ③ ④ ⑤	198 ① ② ③ ④ ⑤
159 ① ② ③ ④ ⑤	169 ① ② ③ ④ ⑤	179 ① ② ③ ④ ⑤	189 ① ② ③ ④ ⑤	199 ① ② ③ ④ ⑤
160 ① ② ③ ④ ⑤	170 ① ② ③ ④ ⑤	180 ① ② ③ ④ ⑤	190 ① ② ③ ④ ⑤	200 ① ② ③ ④ ⑤

EXAMPLES

WRONG
1 ① ⊗ ③ ④ ⑤

WRONG
2 ① ② ③ ④ ⑤

WRONG
3 ① ② ③ ④ ⑤

RIGHT
4 ① ② ③ ● ⑤

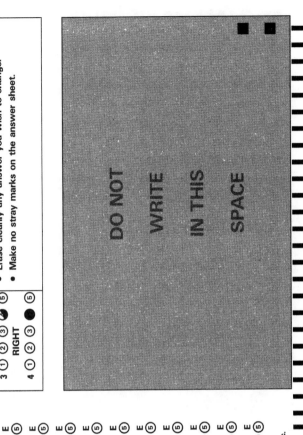

IMPORTANT DIRECTIONS FOR MARKING ANSWERS

- Use #2 pencil only.
- Do NOT use ink or ballpoint pens.
- Make heavy black marks that fill the circle completely.
- Erase cleanly any answer you wish to change.
- Make no stray marks on the answer sheet.

DO NOT WRITE IN THIS SPACE

Trans-Optic® by NCS MPF-4521: 3231302928 Printed in U.S.A.

© 1977 by National Computer Systems, Inc.

EXAM B

1. A breastfeeding mother has been diagnosed with postpartum depression. Her physician contacts you to discuss whether or not she should continue to breastfeed during drug treatment. Your BEST response is:
    a. There are several antidepressant medications that are considered compatible with breastfeeding.
    b. All medications used to treat mental illness are contraindicated during breastfeeding.
    c. Her baby is in great danger and should be kept away from her at all costs.
    d. The hormones of breastfeeding will exacerbate her illness.

2. Which drug property is MOST LIKELY to permit high passage into milk?
    a. High lipid solubility
    b. High pH
    c. Large molecular weight
    d. High protein binding

3. A mother was given 40 mg of a drug with a half-life of 4 hours. How much of the drug is left in her system after 4 half-lives have elapsed?
    a. 20 mg
    b. 10 mg
    c. 5 mg
    d. 2.5 mg

4. Which property of maternal medications INCREASES the amount of the drug that gets to the breastfeeding baby via breastmilk?
    a. short half-life
    b. no active metabolites
    c. high oral absorption
    d. high gut destruction

5. Breastfeeding is usually contraindicated when the mother is taking which category of drug?
    a. antimicrobial
    b. antihypertensive
    c. antineoplastic
    d. antidepressant

Mllk

6. Which mother would have the HIGHEST risk of drug passage into milk?
    a. Sue, whose baby was born at 26 weeks gestation and is now 3 weeks old
    b. Mary, who breastfeeds five times a day and supplements with infant formula
    c. Irene, who had a cesarean birth 2 days ago
    d. Claudia, whose 5-month-old twins are exclusively breastfed

7. Which category of drugs is LEAST LIKELY to remain in breastmilk after the mother stops taking the drug?
    a. marijuana
    b. cocaine
    c. amphetamines
    d. alcohol

8. Which maternal medication is MOST LIKELY to require temporary discarding of the mother's milk?
    a. tetracycline
    b. iodine 131
    c. diazepam
    d. prednisone

9. A mother is concerned because her 3-week-old exclusively breastfed baby suddenly became very fussy in the evenings. Her breastfeeding pattern did not change, and the baby is otherwise healthy. Which recently added item in her diet is MOST LIKELY to be related to her baby's reaction?
    a. lemonade
    b. herb tea
    c. green vegetables
    d. vitamin supplements

10. A breastfeeding mother 6 weeks postbirth tells you "None of your suggestions have worked, and I'm at the end of my rope. I'm a complete failure as a mom!" This situation may be a sign of which of the following conditions?
    a. bipolar disorder
    b. anxiety disorder
    c. postpartum depression
    d. maternal deprivation syndrome

11. Guidelines from the U.S. Centers for Disease Control and Prevention state that health care workers should wear gloves when assisting breastfeeding mothers in which of the following situations?
    a. touching a mother's breast
    b. positioning a baby to breast
    c. helping a mother pump her milk
    d. processing donor human milk

12. Sudden onset of painless, bright red bleeding from the nipple of a mother during the first week postpartum indicates the probable presence of:
    a. breast cancer.
    b. fibrocystic disease.
    c. intraductal papilloma.
    d. nipple tissue breakdown.

13. A pregnant woman who has insulin-dependent diabetes expresses interest in breastfeeding. Your responses should include all of the following EXCEPT:
    a. It may be easier to control your insulin if you breastfeed.
    b. Breastfeeding will help reduce your baby's risk of being diabetic.
    c. It will be more difficult to control your insulin if you breastfeed.
    d. Your colostrum is perfect for your baby, especially in adjusting to extrauterine life.

14. A breastfeeding mother fractured her pelvis and right leg in a car accident. She is in traction and taking pain medications. Her exclusively breastfed 5-month-old baby has never taken a bottle. The MOST helpful action to support this family is:
    a. get her a breastpump so she does not become engorged.
    b. encourage her husband to teach the baby to take milk from a spoon or cup.
    c. help her position the baby for nursing in a way that does not disturb her injuries.
    d. obtain a prescription for birth control pills to dry up her milk.

15. Compared with milk produced by mothers who give birth at full term, preterm milk is higher in which component?
    a. protein
    b. lactose
    c. phosphorus
    d. iron

16. Separating babies from their mothers shortly after birth and caring for them in separate rooms is most likely to result in which of the following?
    a. improved sleep-wake patterns in infants
    b. increased infant stress hormones
    c. more rest for the mother
    d. improved infection control practices

17. A mother complains that her baby is not fitting the feeding schedule recommended by a book she has read. Your BEST response to her is:
    a. It's all right to limit your baby's feeds to 10 minutes per side.
    b. You can give a pacifier to help your baby space out his feeds.
    c. Babies do best when there are no restrictions on length or frequency of breastfeeds.
    d. Giving water between feeds will get him onto a better pattern.

18. John is a 34-week-old premature infant who is being discharged to his parents' care. Breastfeeding discharge teaching correctly includes all of the following EXCEPT:
    a. he should be fed in a position that supports his head, neck and shoulders.
    b. his sucking bursts are regular and rhythmic.
    c. he can adequately reach the lactiferous sinuses.
    d. he needs to be fed every 2 to 3 hours around the clock.

19. A baby who is unable to suck properly is at risk for suboptimal development of all of the following EXCEPT:
    a. orofacial musculature.
    b. gastrointestinal functioning.
    c. urogenital system.
    d. speech and language.

20. Which method of family planning would MOST interfere with breastfeeding?
    a. tubal ligation
    b. progestin-only oral contraceptives
    c. intrauterine devices
    d. natural family planning (periodic abstinence)

21. A healthy, thriving, 10-day-old baby is diagnosed with a bilirubin level of 12 mg/dL (170 μmol/L). The FIRST suggestion for his care should be:
    a. replace most of the breastfeeds with artificial baby milk.
    b. institute phototherapy except during feedings.
    c. continue his 10 to 12 breastfeedings every day.
    d. several sessions undressed in a sunny window.

22. An exclusively breastfed baby is recovering from hernia surgery. Which is the MOST LIKELY breastfeeding pattern for this child?
    a. the same as before the hospitalization
    b. more frequent nursing sessions to quench thirst
    c. longer nursing sessions for the comforting of slow milk flow
    d. less frequent sessions because supply has dropped

23. A mother is concerned that her 1-week-old baby is passing one black, tarry stool per day. The baby nurses about every 3 hours for 15 to 20 minutes. Your FIRST recommendation is:
    a. Relax, the baby is still passing meconium stools.
    b. Have your baby seen by a physician today.
    c. Stop drinking milk because your baby is reacting to the protein.
    d. Begin supplementing because the baby is not getting sufficient fluids.

24. When does the mammary secretory glandular tissue develop?
    a. during puberty
    b. some development occurs with each menstrual period
    c. in the first trimester of pregnancy
    d. during pregnancy and the early weeks postbirth

25. A 16-year-old mother delivered her first baby by cesarean section and sustained significant blood loss requiring a blood transfusion. Four days later, her milk has not yet "come in". The MOST LIKELY reason for delay in onset of copius milk synthesis is:
    a. young age.
    b. cesarean delivery.
    c. first lactation cycle.
    d. significant blood loss.

26. Which is the MOST EFFECTIVE strategy for increasing milk supply?
    a. take fenugreek tea or capsules
    b. drink more fluids
    c. eat more food
    d. hand-express after feeds

27. About an hour after collection, bacterial counts in freshly expressed human milk are lower than immediately after collection. The MOST LIKELY explanation for this is:
    a. the cooler temperature in the container is unsuitable for growth of bacteria.
    b. macrophages in milk are actively phagocytic.
    c. gangliosides in milk disrupt the cell walls of bacteria.
    d. bifidus factor starves the bacteria of nutrients.

28. In a breastfeeding mother, the lactiferous sinuses act as:
    a. secretory glands producing cleansing agents for the areola.
    b. a visual signal for the baby to latch-on.
    c. channels for the milk to flow to the nipple.
    d. milk-secreting glands.

29. The tail of Spence is mammary glandular tissue that:
    a. is only present with supernumerary nipples.
    b. does not produce milk.
    c. extends into the axilla.
    d. is not connected to the breast's duct system.

30. Which of the following is NOT an important function of the nipple-areolar complex in breastfeeding?
    a. visual cue for the baby to latch on
    b. production of lubricants by sebaceous glands
    c. delivery of milk through nipple lumen
    d. nervous system stimulation of the milk-ejection reflex

31. During pregnancy, which characteristic of the breasts is MOST relevant to lactation capacity?
    a. breast growth (size change) during pregnancy
    b. one breast is markedly different in size from the other
    c. colostrum can be expressed from the breasts
    d. tubular shape of the breasts

32. What is the average normal heart rate of a full-term infant?
    a. 80 to 100 beats per minute
    b. 100 to 120 beats per minute
    c. 120 to 160 beats per minute
    d. 160 to 200 beats per minute

33. When during gestation does the mammary ridge form?
    a. 4 to 5 weeks
    b. 14 to 15 weeks
    c. 24 to 25 weeks
    d. 34 to 35 weeks

34. All of the following structures are found in fetal circulation EXCEPT:
    a. ductus venosus
    b. foramen ovale.
    c. ductus arteriosus.
    d. foramen magnum.

35. Pooling or collection of fluid between the skin and cranial bones of the infant's head is called:
    a. caput succedaneum.
    b. cephalhematoma.
    c. periosteal swelling.
    d. hydrocephalus.

36. At what gestational age does the swallowing reflex first appear?
    a. 24 weeks
    b. 26 weeks
    c. 28 weeks
    d. 32 weeks

37. The lymphatic system associated with the lactating breast serves all of the following functions EXCEPT:
    a. drains extracellular fluid from breast tissue
    b. filters bacteria that have entered ducts
    c. provides local responses to infection
    d. supplies lymphocytes present in milk

38. Artificially fed children are at higher risk for all of the following gastrointestinal illnesses EXCEPT:
    a. short gut syndrome
    b. diarrhea
    c. necrotizing enterocolitis (NEC)
    d. Chron's disease

39. Which of the following respiratory conditions is LEAST LIKELY to be related to infant feeding?
    a. otitis media (ear infections)
    b. bronchitis and bronchiolitis
    c. tuberculosis
    d. wheezing/reactive airway disease

40. Viral fragments that appear in mother's milk have all of the following features EXCEPT:
    a. often cause infant illness
    b. act as a "vaccination" against disease
    c. are not whole virus particles
    d. can be killed by heat treatments

41. A disgruntled family files a malpractice suit after you provided lactation consultant services to them. The FIRST thing you should do is:
    a. call an attorney.
    b. contact your professional insurance agent.
    c. talk to the couple to find out why they are upset.
    d. speak to the couple's physician.

42. A mother with influenza asks if she should continue breastfeeding her 5-month-old, exclusively breastfed child. Your responses would include all of the following EXCEPT:
    a. YES, because your milk will quickly contain specific antibodies to lessen the change that your child will get this infection.
    b. YES, because your milk contains white cells that will help your baby fight this infection, if he gets it at all.
    c. YES, because you will get well quicker if you don't have the additional burden of preparing artificial feeds.
    d. YES, because lactation speeds up your own production of antibodies so you won't get as sick.

43. A pregnant woman with many allergies asks about infant feeding. Your BEST response is:
    a. A baby is never allergic to his mother's milk, but he may be sensitive to foods in the mother's diet.
    b. Since many allergic tendencies are inherited, there is nothing you can do to reduce your baby's chances of being allergic.
    c. The hypoallergenic formulas will prevent any allergic reaction in your baby.
    d. Whether you breastfeed or not, you should delay solid foods until 6 months or later to help your baby avoid allergies.

44. When a breastfeeding mother becomes ill:
    a. her milk supply often decreases.
    b. she can transmit many diseases to her baby via her milk.
    c. she can usually continue breastfeeding.
    d. she is likely to be more sick than if she were not breastfeeding.

45. A well-balanced diet with sufficient calories accompanied by early and regular prenatal care significantly reduces the incidence of:
    a. diabetic infants.
    b. low birthweight infants.
    c. maternal gestational diabetes.
    d. lactation failure.

46. Martha is a slender 17-year-old pregnant teenager concerned about eating well enough to help both her body and her new fetus grow. In counseling her, you would consider all of the following EXCEPT:
    a. Take prenatal vitamins every day.
    b. Eat fruits, vegetables and proteins 5 times a day.
    c. Plan your meals and snacks so you eat every few hours.
    d. Plan to gain 15 to 20 pounds by the end of your pregnancy.

47. Which of the following protective components of milk is destroyed by freezing?
    a. lysozyme
    b. T- and B-lymphocytes
    c. secretory IgA
    d. lactoferrin

48. Which hormone in the milk is MOST responsible for antiinflammation activity?
    a. prolactin
    b. prostaglandins
    c. oxytocin
    d. relaxin

49. Prelacteal ritual feeds of butter, herbs, and so on increase the risk of all of the following EXCEPT:
    a. oversupply of milk.
    b. infection with pathogens.
    c. alteration of gut flora.
    d. reduced availability of colostrum.

50. Which milk components causes the stools of exclusively breastfed babies to have a mild, inoffensive, yeast-like odor?
    a. glycopeptides
    b. Candida albicans
    c. phospholipids
    d. bifidus factor

51. Which of the following components of mother's milk varies the MOST with the infant's feeding pattern?
    a. proteins
    b. minerals
    c. fat-soluble vitamins
    d. lactose

52. Some brands of artificial milk produced in the 1980s lacked one essential mineral, causing brain damage in the children who received this product exclusively. Which mineral found in milk was lacking in these products?
    a. sodium
    b. chloride
    c. potassium
    d. calcium

53. Pregnant vegan mothers would need to supplement their plant foods–only diet by taking:
    a. vitamin B12
    b. calcium
    c. fat-soluble vitamins A, D, E, K
    d. iron

54. Carbohydrates in human milk include all of the following EXCEPT:
    a. lactose
    b. oligosaccharides
    c. sucrose
    d. gluconjugates

55. Compared with mature milk, colostrum is:
    a. higher in lactose.
    b. higher in concentration of immunofactors.
    c. higher in volume.
    d. higher in hormones.

56. Which mineral is particularly difficult for the premature (preterm) infant to absorb?
    a. zinc
    b. iron
    c. sodium
    d. chromium

57. Lactose in human milk has all of the following properties EXCEPT:
    a. supply 40% of infant's energy needs
    b. aids absorption of phosphorus and manganese
    c. protects the gastrointestinal tract from pathogens
    d. supports CNS and cognitive development

58. A 4-month-old exclusively breastfed baby feeds about 8 to 10 times per day with 1 to 2 feeds at night. His mother is concerned that she cannot make enough milk because her neighbor had to increase the amount of formula for her baby at 4 months. Your responses to her should include all of the following EXCEPT:
    a. Your baby's feeding pattern indicates that he is ready for solids.
    b. Your baby's milk needs are stable for at least another 2 months.
    c. Your baby is clustering a lot of his milk intake during the daytime, which is normal.
    d. Your baby will take more milk from your breasts if he needs more.

59. A mother is concerned about an "odd smell" in a container of milk that she pumped 2 days ago, and which has been stored in her refrigerator in a closed container. The milk smelled normal when she collected it. The MOST LIKELY cause of this odd smell is:
    a. the protein has been changed by amylase.
    b. the minerals have been changed by bile salt-stimulated lipase.
    c. the fats have been changed by lipase.
    d. the lactose has been changed by lysozyme.

60. Why do the breastfed baby's stools become firmer over time, even before the addition of solid foods?
    a. Casein increases in proportion to whey over time.
    b. There is less liquid in proportion to minerals in the milk over time.
    c. Breastmilk supplies inadequate fluids over time, necessitating adding other drinks.
    d. The baby perspires more, using more of the liquid in milk for metabolism.

61. All of the following components are missing in artificial feeding products EXCEPT:
    a. calcium.
    b. cholesterol.
    c. alpha-lactalbumin.
    d. leukocytes.

62. The standard temperature and time for Holder pasteurization used in human milk banks is:
    a. 56 degrees Celsius for 20 minutes.
    b. 61.4 degrees Celsius for 25 minutes.
    c. 62.5 degrees Celsius for 30 minutes.
    d. 58.6 degrees Celsius for 30 minutes.

63. In the global context, the FOREMOST benefit of using an open cup for feeding a preterm baby who cannot yet breastfeed is:
    a. inexpensive and readily available
    b. low risk of fluid aspiration
    c. fosters appropriate tongue motions
    d. easy to clean

64. The use of teats (artificial nipples) should be avoided for all the following reasons EXCEPT:
    a. Teats can alter the shape of the oral cavity
    b. The liquid can flow too rapidly
    c. The teat may stimulate the palate and trigger suck
    d. Teats can change oralmotor patterning

65. Donor human milk is pasteurized, then frozen, causing which of the following changes?
    a. concentration of lipids
    b. reduction in lactose
    c. no change in Secretory IgA
    d. no change in macrophages

66. When selecting a device to assist breastfeeding, all of the following are principles to follow EXCEPT:
    a. first, do no harm.
    b. select the least expensive device.
    c. use the least intervention for the shortest time.
    d. obtain informed consent from the mother.

67. During a routine examination in her second trimester of pregnancy, a woman is discovered to have nonprotractile nipples. All of the following increase the probability that she will successfully breastfeed EXCEPT:
    a. Instruct her to wear breast shells for increasing amounts of time per day throughout the remainder of her pregnancy.
    b. Teach her appropriate positioning and latch-on techniques.
    c. Encourage her to breastfeed the baby during the first hour after birth, prior to any separation for weighing or measuring.
    d. Encourage her to learn nonpharmaceutical pain relief strategies for labor and birth.

68. The most effective technique for hand-expression of milk is:
    a. compress the breast behind the areola, then slide the fingers toward the nipple.
    b. pinch the base of the nipple.
    c. press deeply at the nipple-areolar juncture.
    d. position fingers at the edge of the areola, press inward, and roll toward the nipple.

69. A full-term baby 13 hours old has not yet been to breast. Your FIRST CHOICE to feed this baby is:
    a. curved-tip syringe.
    b. open cup.
    c. bottle with premie nipple (teat).
    d. put the baby to breast.

70. Which of the following feeding patterns would be MOST LIKELY in a 2-month-old exclusively breastfed baby?
    a. clustering feeds in the late morning
    b. no feeding for 6 to 8 hours at night
    c. Feeds about every 3 to 4 hours during the day and 1 to 2 times at night
    d. 8 to 12 or more feeds spaced throughout the 24-hour day

71. 12-hour-old Rose was born after 15 hours of hard labor and pushing, with forceps and vacuum extractor, deep suctioned for meconium above the cords, and molded cranium and puncture mark from an internal monitor probe. Her mother is anxious to bond and breastfeed within the first hour after delivery. Rose is very sleepy. Your FIRST intervention will be to:
    a. bring Rose horizontally to her mother's breast level.
    b. rub Rose's face with a cold wash cloth.
    c. pull Rose's chin down for a latch on.
    d. place Rose skin to skin with her mother and turn down the lights.

72. A 5-month-old exclusively breastfed baby is suddenly hospitalized for treatment of a cardiac abnormality. The mother is told she must stop breastfeeding because the baby's intake and output need to be carefully measured. Of the following options, which is least likely to disrupt the breastfeeding relationship and provide accurate information on intake?
    a. mother expresses her milk and gives it by an alternative feeding device
    b. weigh the baby before and after feeds
    c. weigh the mother before and after feeds
    d. carefully count the baby's swallows and record duration of breastfeeding

73. When revising or creating policies relating to breastfeeding, which of the following provides the WEAKEST evidence for the policy?
    a. systematic reviews and meta-analyses
    b. randomized controlled trials
    c. cross-sectional surveys
    d. case reports

74. When doing a review of the literature for a research study, which sources are MOST IMPORTANT to include?
    a. review articles which analyze several studies
    b. textbooks that explain basic concepts
    c. peer-reviewed journal report of research, written by the researcher
    d. lectures given at large conferences by well-known speakers

75. You think you are seeing a certain phenomenon in your clients. In order to study this more thoroughly, you might do any of the following EXCEPT:
    a. observational study
    b. qualitiative survey
    c. case reports
    d. clinical trial

76. A researcher is studying breastfeeding incidence in two neighboring community prenatal clinics. In one clinic, a new videotape is used to teach breastfeeding; the other continues to use an older videotape. At the follow-up, both clinics report similar increases in breastfeeding initiation. The MOST LIKELY reason for this is:
    a. all instructional videotapes are equivalent.
    b. the Hawthorne effect.
    c. changing the videotape had no effect.
    d. the Nedelsky effect.

77. The American Academy of Pediatrics and the Innocenti Declaration recommend exclusive breastfeeding for what length of time?
    a. 4 months
    b. 6 months
    c. 12 months
    d. Infant self-weaning

78. A mother has begun breastfeeding successfully and is leaving the hospital with her 4-day-old son today. Your BEST action is to:
    a. call her in a week to see how things are going.
    b. refer her to a local mother support group.
    c. enroll her in a food supplement program in case she needs infant formula.
    d. make sure she has a written pamphlet on breastfeeding.

79. The Innocenti Declaration contains all of the following Operational Targets EXCEPT:
    a. appointment of a national breastfeeding coordinator and committee.
    b. adherence to the Ten Steps to Successful Breastfeeding by every maternity facility.
    c. implementation of the International Code of Marketing of Breastmilk Substitutes.
    d. passage of legislation protecting a mother's right to breastfeed in public.

80. Health policies that are affected by breastfeeding rates include all of the following EXCEPT:
    a. food security.
    b. environmental protection.
    c. reduction in family violence.
    d. economic development.

81. Safe motherhood initiatives include breastfeeding because it protects women's health in all of the following ways EXCEPT:
    a. reduced postpartum bleeding.
    b. reduced risk of reproductive cancers.
    c. reduce postpartum fertility.
    d. reduced libido during breastfeeding.

82. The International Code of Marketing of Breast-Milk Substitutes applies to all of the following products EXCEPT:
    a. breast pumps.
    b. infant formula.
    c. feeding bottles and teats.
    d. weaning foods.

83. Which of the following situations DOES NOT require written documentation?
    a. phone calls from clients
    b. bedside contacts with clients in hospital
    c. clinic or office visits when the primary care physician also sees the client
    d. telephone inquiries about business hours or prices

84. All of the following collaborations are appropriate for an IBCLC EXCEPT:
    a. providing newsletters from the local mother support group to mothers in your practice.
    b. Working closely with a Registered Dietitian in the case of a baby diagnosed with phenylketonuria (PKU).
    c. consulting with a surgeon before you provide breastfeeding assistance to the mother of a newborn with an unrepaired cleft palate.
    d. discussing a feverish mother's inflamed breast with her physician to develop an appropriate care plan that preserves breastfeeding.

85. Which of the following actions by an IBCLC is NOT within the LC scope of practice?
    a. examining a breastfeeding mother's breast.
    b. developing supplementing policies for the NICU.
    c. dispensing and instructing on the use of breast pumps.
    d. advising a mother that prescribed medication is safe to use during breastfeeding.

86. A mother tells you that the pediatrician has recommended that she give artificial baby milk after each breastfeeding to her slow-gaining 9-week-old infant. What would NOT be an appropriate initial response?
    a. Offer alternative suggestions to frequent complementation.
    b. Refer her to a different pediatrician.
    c. Refer her to a breastfeeding support group.
    d. Give information on how to provide complementary feeding without compromising breastfeeding.

87. In order to minimize your legal risk when practicing as a lactation consultant, it is MOST important for you to:
    a. keep accurate financial records.
    b. get detailed information about families from their other health care providers.
    c. establish a respectful rapport with open communication.
    d. accept their insurance payment plan.

88. A mother of newborn twins asks whether to feed her babies separately or together. Your BEST response is:
    a. Let's see which works best for you.
    b. Separately is better so you can focus on one at a time.
    c. Together is better to save you time.
    d. Feed them together to get their feeding patterns synchronized.

89. You have been working with a mother who describes excruciating pain every time her baby's mouth touches her breast, even if he does not latch on and breastfeed. You have ruled out injury, infections, and other causes of nipple pain, and her nipples are not reddened or irritated. You should NEXT consider whether the mother has:
    a. a history of any kind of abuse.
    b. no interest in breastfeeding.
    c. a low pain threshold.
    d. allergies.

90. A mother asks you to help her write a birth plan that will optimize her success with breastfeeding. Her plan should include all of the following EXCEPT:
    a. place of birth where she feels safest.
    b. choice of companions and family members.
    c. access to furniture, hot tub, and equipment that encourages motion and posture changes.
    d. professional attendant who will give her specific directions during her labor.

91. A cultural attitude that emphasizes the sexual nature of breasts is most LIKELY associated with:
    a. harassment for breastfeeding in public.
    b. increased breast augmentation surgery.
    c. mothers enjoying the attention created by larger breasts during lactation.
    d. conflicts in custody disputes involving breastfeeding babies.

92. Breastfeeding mothers are LEAST LIKELY to experience which of the following psychosocial effects?
    a. calming effect of lactational hormones
    b. enhanced fulfillment of their maternal role
    c. less work time lost because of children's illness
    d. higher blood pressure because of the metabolic demands of breastfeeding

93. A mother in Western industrialized cultures is MOST likely to continue breastfeeding past 1 year if which of the following people support this idea?
    a. her male partner
    b. her father
    c. her doctor
    d. her sister

94. Breastfeeding as an oral function of the baby involves all of the following EXCEPT:
    a. sense of taste and smell of milk.
    b. oral gratification as described by Freud.
    c. tactile sensation of breast filling the infant's mouth.
    d. inability of infant to control shape of breast.

95. Which statement BEST describes the role of the father and the exclusively breastfed baby?
    a. Breastfeeding increases the father's jealousy of the mother-baby relationship.
    b. Fathers of breastfed babies miss out on the opportunity to bond during feeding.
    c. Breastfeeding is not a barrier to father-child bonding.
    d. The baby may attempt to feed from the father's breasts.

96. A mother with a 5-day-old infant repeatedly requests "rules" for how many times a day she should feed her baby. This behavior is typical of which stage of maternal role acquisition?
    a. anticipatory
    b. formal
    c. informal
    d. personal

97. A 6-month-old baby, sitting at the family dinner table, begins reaching for food. Which statement BEST describes the reason for this behavior?
    a. The baby is developmentally ready for solid food.
    b. The mother's milk supply is no longer adequate.
    c. The baby is just imitating and will not be ready for family foods for some time.
    d. The baby is jealous because everyone else is eating real food.

98. What event triggers Lactogenesis II (onset of copious milk secretion)?
     a. stimulation from baby at breast.
     b. drop in progesterone from placenta separation.
     c. rise in oxytocin from uterine contractions.
     d. change in blood pH when umbilical cord is cut.

99. A mother calls $5\frac{1}{2}$ weeks after delivering a full term infant. She tells you she is losing her milk because her breasts are soft and her infant no longer seems content for 2 hours after feedings. He cries frequently and puts his fists to his mouth 45 minutes after feeding. The MOST LIKELY cause for the situation she describes is:
     a. her infant is experiencing a growth spurt.
     b. offering bottles is interfering with breastmilk production.
     c. the development of colic in her infant.
     d. her body is adapting well to her baby's demand for milk.

100. A 2-day-old baby feeds from one breast for about 25 minutes, then falls asleep and releases the breast. A few minutes later, he wakes and feeds on the second breast for about 10 minutes, then falls asleep and releases the breast. The MOST LIKELY explanation for this behavior is:
     a. The mother does not yet have enough milk to satisfy the baby.
     b. The baby is not latched deeply onto the breast.
     c. The baby is sleepy and poorly coordinated as a result of labor medications.
     d. This is a normal pattern for a baby this age .

101. At which ages/stages are babies MOST likely to self-wean?
     a. Under 12 months
     b. 12 to 18 months
     c. 2 to $2\frac{1}{2}$ years
     d. 3 to 4 years

102. A mother has been feeding her baby on a rigid schedule for several months on the advice of friends. Her child is now underweight, appears anxious, and cries frequently. She strongly desires to continue breastfeeding. Your BEST recommendation is:
     a. Increase the amount of solid food he is getting.
     b. Pump your milk between feeds to keep up your supply.
     c. Add artificial milk to his feeds so he can stay on this schedule.
     d. Discontinue scheduled feeds and feed the baby whenever he is hungry.

103. After an unmedicated labor and birth, how soon is a baby MOST LIKELY to be able and ready to breastfeed?
    a. within the first 5 minutes
    b. within the first hour
    c. at approximately 6 hours
    d. by 12 hours

104. At what developmental age is self-feeding MOST LIKELY to begin?
    a. 3 months
    b. 6 months
    c. 9 months
    d. 12 months

105. For an 18-month-old child, breastfeeding is LEAST significant as a source of:
    a. calories.
    b. immunities.
    c. comfort.
    d. bonding.

106. A 5-month-old breastfed baby's mother feels that she should learn how to sleep for at least 8 straight hours at night. Your BEST response to her is:
    a. at this age, she needs frequent contact with you for reassurance that you are there.
    b. she is old enough to self-soothe now.
    c. she has already learned how to manipulate you; you had better train her to sleep.
    d. now that she is not a newborn, you do not need to respond right away when she cries.

107. A researcher plans to study the effect of giving breastfeeding mothers an herbal preparation to increase milk supply. The mothers are all from the same community, and their babies are in the same age range. Which of the following is the DEPENDENT variable in this study?
    a. use of the herbal preparation *independent*
    b. milk volume intake of the babies
    c. amount of milk pumped
    d. use of a placebo preparation

108. A mother and her breastfeeding toddler twins are likely to experience all of the following EXCEPT:
    a.   mutual enjoyment of breastfeeding.
    b.   sibling rivalry for the breast.
    c.   playfulness between children during feeds.
    d.   higher risk of milk stasis.

109. All of the following practices might suggest that a health care provider is supportive of breastfeeding EXCEPT:
    a.   breastfeeding texts on office shelves.
    b.   breastfeeding gift packs that include formula samples.
    c.   Lactation Consultant on staff.
    d.   list of mother support groups provided to all clients.

110. A pregnant woman contracted chickenpox a short time ago. The lesions are now completely crusted over, and she is in labor. The most appropriate action to take when she gives birth is:
    a.   separate her from the baby until she is noninfectious.
    b.   allow her to hold, but not breastfeed her baby.
    c.   separate her from the baby but feed her expressed milk to the baby.
    d.   help her breastfeed immediately after birth with 24-hour rooming-in.

111. Which is the LEAST important function of colostrum?
    a.   coats the immature gut and prevents adherence of pathogens
    b.   provides high-calorie food for energy
    c.   blocks transmission of allergens
    d.   white cells actively attack bacteria

112. The LEAST LIKELY cause for a mother's nipples to be cracked and bleeding on the second postpartum day is:
    a.   baby has anklyoglossia
    b.   baby is latching only onto the nipple
    c.   mother has unusually fragile nipple skin
    d.   mother is feeding her baby every 2 hours for 30 minutes each

113. Which of the following statements BEST describes the Babinski reflex?
    a.   grasp object when palm is stimulated
    b.   turn mouth toward source of stimulation
    c.   bear partial weight of body while standing on flat surface
    d.   flare toes when sole of foot is stimulated

114. A pregnant mother is HIV positive but otherwise healthy. She wants to breastfeed her baby. The FIRST THING you should do is:
    a. tell her breastfeeding is contraindicated for HIV positive mothers.
    b. tell her breastfeeding is not contraindicated.
    c. have her talk to her doctor.
    d. share recommendations of the CDC, UNICEF, and WHO.

115. A pregnant woman has heard that letting epidural anesthesia wear off prior to delivery will avoid anesthesia-related breastfeeding problems. You should tell her all of the following EXCEPT:
    a. drugs can take much longer to clear the baby's system, so there is still a possible breastfeeding risk with this approach.
    b. the combination of drugs used in epidural anesthesia makes it difficult to determine which medications cause breastfeeding problems.
    c. epidural anesthesia has minimal or no effect on the baby regardless of how long before delivery it is administered.
    d. epidural anesthesia increases the likelihood of other birth interventions that can affect breastfeeding.

116. A research report indicates that a sample of breastfed infants had no differences in illness rates than a comparable sample of artificially fed infants. While reading this report, the MOST IMPORTANT point to look for is:
    a. the type of study used.
    b. operational definitions.
    c. the sample used.
    d. the review of the literature.

117. Which of the following citations is a PRIMARY reference or source?
    a. DeCoopman, JM. *Pacifier Use in Breastfed Infants: Review and Recommendations.* (Masters' Thesis). Ann Arbor: University of Michigan, 1996.
    b. Als H, Lester BM, Tronick E and Brazelton TB. Manual for the assessment of preterm infants' behavior (AFPB). In Fitzgerald JE, Lester BM, Jogman MW, eds. *Theory and Research in Behavioral Pediatrics,* Vol 1, New York: Plenum, 1982, 64-133.
    c. Fildes V. *Breasts, Bottles and Babies: A History of Infant Feeding.* Edinburgh: Edinburgh University Press, 1986.
    d. Aarts C, Hornell A, Kylberg E, et al. Breastfeeding patterns in relation to thumb sucking and pacifier use. *Pediatrics* 1999; 104(4).

118. A mother of a fussy, gassy baby has been drinking 10 glasses of milk per day on her doctor's recommendation. Your FIRST action would be:
    a. Encourage her to follow her doctor's dietary advice.
    b. Take a thorough history including allergy and food sensitivity in the family.
    c. Tell her that 6 to 8 glasses of any liquid is adequate during lactation.
    d. Tell her that consumption of dairy products is not related to her baby's symptoms.

119. When selecting a drug to be given to a breastfeeding woman, which of the following drug properties is MOST IMPORTANT to consider?
    a. absorption from the GI tract
    b. protein binding
    c. milk/plasma ratio
    d. pediatric half-life

120. The most important determinant of drug penetration into milk is the mother's:
    a. plasma level.
    b. weight.
    c. blood type.
    d. milk storage capacity.

121. A mother complains of raw, inflamed skin on both areolas. Her infant is teething, has recently started solid foods and is taking an antibiotic for strep throat. The MOST LIKELY cause of the areolar irritation is:
    a. allergic reaction to a food the baby consumed.
    b. allergic reaction to the medication being given to her infant.
    c. psoriasis that was exacerbated by the infant's saliva.
    d. bacterial infection of the nipple skin.

122. A mother is concerned because her areola is over 4 inches (10 cm) in diameter, and drops of milk appear on the areola when her milk lets down. How will this affect her ability to breastfeed?
    a. The areola is too large to fit completely inside the baby's mouth.
    b. The misplaced milk duct openings will make it difficult for her baby to latch.
    c. Very large areolas are associated with milk oversupply.
    d. Her breasts are normal—she should easily be able to breastfeed.

123. The mother of this baby complains of itching, burning pain in her nipples. The recommendation MOST LIKELY to resolve her pain is:
    a. Breastfeed for frequent short periods of time.
    b. Wear nipple shields during breastfeeding for one week.
    c. Mother and baby are treated with antifungal medication.
    d. Boil all the baby's pacifiers.

124. The cause of this toddler's dental condition is LEAST LIKELY to be due to:
    a. high intake of sweetened foods.
    b. lack of tooth-brushing.
    c. congenital enamel defects.
    d. unrestricted breastfeeding at night.

125. Any breastfeeding difficulties experienced by this infant are MOST LIKELY related to:
    a. fetal alcohol syndrome.
    b. congenital hypothyroidism.
    c. Down syndrome.
    d. Pierre Robin syndrome.

126. Which of the following sensations is this mother MOST LIKELY to be experiencing?
    a. comfort during and between feeds
    b. systemic fever and chills
    c. deep, aching breast pain
    d. burning, stinging, or itching of both nipples/areolas

127. The nipple damage shown in this picture is MOST LIKELY due to:
    a. poor positioning at breast.
    b. bacterial or fungal infection.
    c. tongue-tied baby.
    d. overuse of a breast pump.

128. All of the following are appropriate actions for this mother's situation EXCEPT:
    a. Advise her to stop breastfeeding on this breast.
    b. Assist her to express milk from this breast thoroughly every few hours.
    c. Encourage her to rest and continue breastfeeding on the other breast.
    d. Support her taking any prescribed antibiotics.

129.   Which is the MOST LIKELY cause of the condition pictured?
    a.   baby is teething
    b.   allergic response to laundry soap used to wash bra
    c.   suction too high on breastpump
    (d.)   baby has a bacterial infection of the mouth

130.   This baby just came off the breast. What is this mother MOST LIKELY feeling?
    (a.)   pinching nipple pain
    b.   aching breast pain
    c.   relaxation and sleepiness
    d.   relief that the baby fed well

131.   This mother is one week postpartum and experiencing nipple pain. The MOST LIKELY explanation is:
    a.   inversion in the center of the tip is rubbing on the baby's palate.
    (b.)   large, fibrous nipple is being compressed by baby's mouth.
    c.   edema of the nipple from baby's vigorous suck.
    d.   primary engorgement.

132.   What is your BEST recommendation for the condition pictured?
    a.   rub cocoa butter into the sore area
    b.   rinse with hydrogen peroxide several times a day
    (c.)   use a dressing that is designed for moist wound healing on the wound
    d.   apply vitamin E oil to the nipple tip

133.   What is the MOST LIKELY condition shown in this picture?
    (a.)   unpigmented areola
    b.   poison ivy
    c.   normal breast
    d.   fungal infection

134.   This 6-day-old baby has been nursing about every 4 hours during the day and once at night, and has not regained birthweight. The mother has asked for help breastfeeding. At the time this picture was taken, he had been sleeping since his last feed ended 3 hours ago. Your recommendations to the mother should include all of the following EXCEPT:
    a.   Try giving him some expressed breastmilk with a spoon right now.
    b.   Please undress him so we can check his weight.
    (c.)   Take him to his physician's office or an emergency room immediately.
    d.   Let's see what he does at breast, even while he's sleepy.

135. What is the MOST LIKELY reason this mother is experiencing pain in her left axilla?
    a. severe postpartum engorgement
    b. lactogenesis II in axillary mammary tissue
    c. allergic reaction to a new deodorant
    d. overuse strain of the pectoral muscles

136. What could you do to DECREASE this baby's risk of SIDS?
    a. Move the mattress away from the unused fireplace.
    b. Put the baby in a crib.
    c. Give the baby a pacifier.
    d. Roll the baby onto her back.

137. What correlates most closely with the age of the child pictured?
    a. will no longer take a pacifier
    b. highest risk of SIDS
    c. ability to roll over
    d. highest risk of otitis media

138. This mother complains of nipple pain while pumping. The MOST LIKELY cause is:
    a. she has a fungal infection on her nipples.
    b. the pump flange is not centered over her nipple.
    c. the pressure on the pump is too high.
    d. her lower hand is pulling the breast away from the pump.

139. This breastfeeding mother says that this condition appeared when her baby was about 4 months old. Which is the LEAST LIKELY cause of the condition shown?
    a. atopic dermatitis
    b. fungal infection
    c. eczema
    d. psoriasis

140. This picture was taken 3 hours after the baby fed on this breast. The condition pictured is MOST LIKELY:
    a. infectious mastitis in the upper, outer quadrant.
    b. galactocele on the lateral side (toward the mother's arm).
    c. normal postfeed breast fullness.
    d. edema caused by milk statis.

141. This mother's baby keeps bobbing on and off the breast, and can't quite latch on. The FIRST action she should take is:
    a. place a nipple shield over her nipple.
    b. let her baby suck on her finger to calm him.
    c. express some milk to soften the breast.
    d. burp him first before trying again.

142. What would you do NEXT to help this baby breastfeed?
    a. Immediately put him to breast while he is alert.
    b. Put him under a radiant warmer for 2 hours to stabilize his temperature.
    c. Put him upright on his mother's bare chest, covered with a loose blanket.
    d. Swaddle him tightly with a small blanket to contain extraneous movements.

143. What neurodevelopmental state is this baby in?
    a. drowsy
    b. quiet alert
    c. active alert
    d. REM sleep

144. Upon seeing this 14-day-old infant, the FIRST question you would ask the mother about her own health status is:
    a. Are you getting enough rest?
    b. Are you eating a well-balanced diet?
    c. Do you have a fever?
    d. What color and quantity is your vaginal discharge?

145. This picture was taken immediately after a feed ended. Which statement MOST LIKELY describes the preceding feed?
    a. Baby was poorly latched.
    b. Baby was deeply latched.
    c. Baby effectively transferred milk.
    d. Baby fed well, then self-detached.

146. This mother tells you that her child loves the device pictured and sleeps best this way. The MOST LIKELY reason for this is:
    a. the child has become too dependent because of prolonged breastfeeding.
    b. overuse of the baby carrier has delayed the child's ability to sleep alone.
    c. the mother is using her child to meet her own needs for companionship.
    d. this is normal behavior for a child this age.

147. This 4-week-old exclusively breastfed baby was 6 lbs, 3 oz at birth. The MOST LIKELY reason for her appearance at this age is:
    a. her mother's milk is too high in fat.
    b. she is taking steroid drugs for a medical condition.
    c. mother feeds her on cue, 24 hours a day, without a pacifier.
    d. mother's milk is too high in lactose.

148. The asymmetry of this woman's breasts is MOST LIKELY due to:
    a. normal development.
    b. inadequate milk supply in the smaller breast.
    c. insufficient glandular tissue in the smaller breast.
    d. hypermastia in the larger breast.

149. Which structure in this baby's mouth is MOST LIKELY to cause a breastfeeding problem?
    a. alveolar gum ridge
    b. philtrim
    c. lingual frenulum
    d. short tongue

150. This child's mother tried unsuccessfully to breastfeed, and her child now has difficulty eating. The MOST LIKELY reason is that this child has:
    a. anklyoglossia.
    b. macroglossia.
    c. microglossia.
    d. micrognathia.

151. What is the MOST ACCURATE description of this nipple shape?
    a. normal
    b. flat
    c. conical
    d. inverted

152. This mother wants to know if her breasts and nipples are normal. Which of the following is the LEAST APPROPRIATE response?
    a. Your breasts are entirely normal.
    b. Your nipple is slightly retracted.
    c. Your areola is slightly narrow in diameter.
    d. Your large nipple will likely be a problem for your baby.

153. This mother has a 2-week-old baby who has difficulty attaching to her smaller breast, has been fussy after feeds, and has not regained birthweight. She claims that she does not have enough milk. The MOST LIKELY cause of this situation is:
    a. the mother is not feeding her baby frequently enough.
    b. the smaller breast has insufficient glandular tissue.
    c. the baby is attached incorrectly to the breast.
    d. the baby is sensitive to an allergen in his mother's milk.

154. This mother is currently breastfeeding a 2-year-old. The condition pictured on her areola is MOST LIKELY:
    a. herpes (viral) infection.
    b. wounds from the child biting.
    c. normal Montgomery glands.
    d. urticaria (hives).

155. This mother is concerned about the appearance of her nipples. Your BEST response is:
    a. You probably have a thrush infection.
    b. A bacterial infection is a possibility.
    c. Don't breastfeed until the herpes lesion heals.
    d. Your breast is entirely normal.

156. The condition pictured appeared on day 4 postpartum. The mother might be experiencing a similar phenomenon in any of the following locations EXCEPT:
    a. near the umbilicus.
    b. upper, inner arm.
    c. groin.
    d. outer thigh.

157. What is the LEAST LIKELY explanation for the color of this milk, which was collected on day 5?
    a. The mother is taking prenatal vitamins containing beta carotene.
    b. The milk contains pus from the mother's breast infection.
    c. Transitional milk normally contains significant amounts of colostrum.
    d. The mother had carrots and sweet potatoes for dinner last night.

158. The condition pictured appeared suddenly several days ago, when the baby began spending several hours daily in a day care facility. The MOST LIKELY cause of the condition pictured is:
     a. the baby's mother recently began taking an antibiotic.
     b. the baby recently ingested two bottles of artificial baby milk.
     c. the baby shared teething toys with other children.
     d. the baby's diaper does not get changed often enough.

159. Which of the following is the MOST LIKELY cause of the condition pictured?
     a. cold temperature in the room
     b. supplements of cow-milk based formula
     c. supplements of rice cereal
     d. baby recently had a tetanus immunization

160. What is the AVERAGE volume of milk consumed over 24 hours by a breastfed baby of this age?
     a. 240 to 300 ml (8 to 10 oz) per day
     b. 480 to 540 ml (16 to 18 oz) per day
     c. 720 to 780 ml (24 to 26 oz) per day
     d. 900 to 960 ml (30 to 32 oz) per day

161. At this stage of lactation, all of the following components of human milk are increased over newborn-period EXCEPT:
     a. lyzozyme.
     b. casein.
     c. fats.
     d. serotonin.

162. This mother has been using a piece of equipment to help resolve her breastfeeding problem. Which is the MOST LIKELY product that she used?
     a. nipple shields
     b. breast shells
     c. bottle teat placed over her nipple
     d. breast pump

163. This mother's baby is 4 days old. She is MOST LIKELY using this equipment to:
     a. remove excess milk.
     b. stimulate the breast to make milk.
     c. correct inverted nipples.
     d. prevent mastitis.

164. Advantages of using this alternative feeding technique include all of the following EXCEPT:
    a. easy to clean the equipment
    b. can pace to baby's ability
    c. prevents nipple confusion
    d. inexpensive

165. This breastfeeding mother is being treated for a fungal (candida) infection on her nipples. You should recommend all of the following EXCEPT:
    a. Boil all baby's teething objects, including this toothbrush.
    b. Wash hands before and after contact with baby's mouth or diaper area.
    c. Wash bras in hot water with a small amount of bleach.
    d. Use a nipple shield during feeds to prevent transfer to baby.

166. The MOST IMPORTANT action to take in helping this mother breastfeed is:
    a. Have her wear a nipple shield during feedings.
    b. Hand-express milk before feeds to soften the large nipple area.
    c. Help the baby latch on to the breast deeply, taking the entire nipple-areola complex into his mouth.
    d. Apply an antifungal preparation to the nipples after every feed.

167. This baby attaches to the breast, feeds steadily and comfortably for about 17 minutes, then releases the breast. Which of the following actions IS MOST APPROPRIATE for mother?
    a. Use your other hand to support your breast during feeds.
    b. Bring your arm closer to your baby's neck.
    c. No suggestions.
    d. Pull your baby's legs closer to you.

168. This feeding technique and equipment are possible solutions for all of the following situations EXCEPT:
    a. increased sensory input to palate.
    b. skin-to-mouth contact.
    c. prevention of nipple confusion/flow preference.
    d. immediately after cleft palate repair.

169. Appropriate treatments for this condition include all of the following EXCEPT:
    a. cabbage leaf compresses.
    b. hot compresses.
    c. cold compresses.
    d. gentle massage.

170. What, if anything, would you suggest to this mother regarding her baby's position and latch?
    a. Everything looks good.
    (b) Try uncurling his lower lip with your finger.
    c. Tickle his feet so he wakes up during feeds.
    d. Press down on your breast so his nostrils are clear.

171. A mother and baby are MOST LIKELY to prefer the underarm (vertical) position for which of the following reasons?
    (a) infant has greater head stability
    b. stronger let-down reflex
    c. less chance of plugged milk ducts
    d. reduces infant colic

172. This mother's breast is very hard and painful. All of the following interventions are appropriate EXCEPT:
    a. Document her history leading up to this situation.
    b. Wearing gloves, assess the degree of milk stasis in the breast tissue.
    (c) Clean the incision and surrounding skin with an antiseptic solution.
    d. Gently teach or assist in expressing milk from the injured breast.

173. What is the mother of this baby MOST LIKELY to be feeling?
    (a) itching, stinging, burning nipple pain
    b. deep aching pain in her breast
    c. comfortable breasts and nipples
    d. sharp, stabbing pain after and between feedings

174. This breastfeeding baby might demonstrate any of the following feeding patterns EXCEPT:
    a. self-feed with pincer grasp.
    b. sip liquids from an open cup.
    (c) self-wean from the breast.
    d. breastfeed 8 to 16 times a day.

175. What is the most appropriate documentation of the appearance of this woman's breast?
    a. red circular area on the areola near the nipple margin
    (b) red lesion $\frac{1}{2}$ inch (1 cm) diameter on the areola at the 7 o'clock position
    c. bacterial infection on the areolar skin in the lower, outer quadrant
    d. painful nipples with reddened area below the nipple base

176.   What would be the MOST appropriate use for this technique?
    a.   baby less than 24 hours old and not yet nursing
    b.   baby 6 months old refusing solid foods
    c.   baby has poor suck, and mother's nipples are damaged
    d.   supplementing a 4-day-old baby who is 7% below birthweight

177.   This mother says she has been hand-expressing her milk as shown in the picture. Which is the MOST LIKELY result of her using the technique pictured?
    a.   Milk is easily expressed.
    b.   Little or no milk flows.
    c.   The areola is bruised.
    d.   The nipple and areola become more elastic.

178.   This baby is 2 weeks old and still under his birth weight. The mother's nipples are cracked, scabbed, and painful. Feeds are 30 to 45 minutes long every 2 hours round the clock. The mother is exhausted. The FIRST recommendation you would give to his mother is:
    a.   Have the baby's pediatrician or dentist evaluate his frenulum.
    b.   He's obviously upset—give him a pacifier to calm him before trying to breastfeed.
    c.   Are you willing to try feeding him some expressed milk in a cup?
    d.   Go to bed with him and try nursing lying down in a darkened room.

179.   This condition has persisted for 2½ months. What is the MOST HELPFUL action you could take for this mother?
    a.   thoroughly examine the baby's nursing technique at breast
    b.   refer her to a dermatologist for further evaluation
    c.   provide her with moist wound healing preparations
    d.   recommend she pump or express and feed the baby with a device

180.   What is this mother doing?
    a.   expressing colostrum
    b.   pinch test
    c.   everting her retracting nipple
    d.   nipple rolling to firm the tip

181.   The mother in this picture is preparing to breastfeed her baby. Your FIRST suggestion would be:
    a.   Great technique to firm your nipples!
    b.   Move your hand back behind the areola to support your breast.
    c.   Place the nipple tip in the baby's mouth.
    d.   Pinching your nipple can injure the tissue.

182. This technique might be used for all of the following EXCEPT:
    a. massaging a plugged nipple pore.
    b. firming the nipple tip before feeding.
    c. expressing milk.
    d. increasing tissue elasticity.

183. This mother is 4 days postpartum. Your FIRST advice to assist her in breastfeeding should be:
    a. Support your breast and bring the baby to you.
    b. Use warm compresses to soften the areola.
    c. Use cool compresses to reduce edema.
    d. Express some milk to soften the breast.

184. Which conclusion can be drawn from Chart 1?
    a. Baby A will always be smaller than baby D.
    b. Baby B gained weight faster than the others.
    c. Baby C is failing to thrive.
    d. Baby D gained the most weight in 1 month.

185. At the age shown, what is the MOST APPROPRIATE recommendation for this child's nutrition?
    a. exclusive breastfeeding around the clock
    b. breastfeeding with added carbohydrates
    c. breastfeeding with complementary family foods
    d. breastfeeding supplemented with infant formula

186. This child's imitative behavior suggests which of the following?
    a. latent homosexuality
    b. normal behavior modeling
    c. deviant behavior
    d. precocious sexuality

187. Your neighbor requests information on allowing her children to nap together. Your BEST response is:
    a. The children look very cute when they are asleep.
    b. The infant is in extreme danger from overlying.
    c. Children should learn to sleep in their own beds.
    d. Siblings sleeping together is common around the world.

188. This pregnant mother calls and complains of tender nipples and lower milk supply. Your BEST response is:
    a. It's best if you start weaning your daughter; she's nursed long enough already.
    b. See your doctor about the sudden onset nipple pain—it might be thrush.
    c. Drink fenugreek tea to increase your milk supply.
    d. What you're experiencing is common for women who are pregnant and still breastfeeding. How do you feel about continuing to breastfeed?

189. This baby's weight gain and development are normal. What is the FIRST question you would ask the mother?
    a. Do you use this position at all feeds?
    b. Is your baby sleeping through the night yet?
    c. How is breastfeeding going for you?
    d. Have your menstrual periods returned?

190. In this situation, which aspect of maternal infant bonding is most likely to occur FIRST?
    a. mother bonds with the "unit"
    b. mother bonds with the firstborn
    c. mother bonds with the lastborn
    d. mother has delayed bonding with all

191. Which of the following is the LEAST LIKELY condition pictured?
    a. galactocele
    b. areolar edema
    c. abscess
    d. milk stasis

192. Breastfeeding behaviors common to a child of this age include all of the following EXCEPT:
    a. playfulness at breast.
    b. ability to breastfeed while mother is engaging in other activities.
    c. persistent biting.
    d. breastfeeding at night.

193. A baby of this age is likely to show all of the following behaviors EXCEPT:
    a. hands frequently open
    b. follows light to midline
    c. reaches for object
    d. differentiated cries and sounds

194. The nursing baby in this picture has not yet shown any interest in eating any family foods. Your responses would include all of the following EXCEPT:
    a. His growth is faltering, so you'll need to try harder to get him to eat family food.
    b. Exclusive breastfeeding for longer than 6 months is within normal growth patterns.
    c. With your family history of allergies, it's not surprising that he's avoiding other foods.
    d. Your other child is probably distracting him at mealtimes.

195. Of the following conditions, which is LEAST LIKELY to result in this pattern of growth?
    a. Down syndrome
    b. exclusive breastfeeding
    c. tongue-tied baby
    d. cystic fibrosis

196. This breastfeeding behavior is MOST likely to occur at which age?
    a. 5 to 6 months
    b. 7 to 12 months
    c. 12 to 18 months
    d. 18 to 24 months

197. The likely consequences of this behavior include all of the following EXCEPT:
    a. baby receives up to 30% of calories at night.
    b. increased risk of baby smothering.
    c. reduced risk of early weaning.
    d. reduced risk of pregnancy.

198. This exclusively breastfed baby's weight has dropped a bit on the NCHS standardized growth charts that were in use prior to 2000. Her development in other areas is completely normal to advanced, and she is content and happy most of the time. The MOST LIKELY reason for this apparent growth faltering is:
    a. the mother's milk is too low in fat.
    b. the baby is physiologically ready for solid foods.
    c. breastfeeding requires extra energy intake at this age.
    d. breastfed babies tend to be leaner than artificially fed babies at this age.

199. Which statement are you MOST LIKELY to hear from the mother of this child?
    a. My baby has been weaning herself—she's down to three nursings a day.
    b. She just started sleeping through the night without nursing.
    c. She's been so clingy lately—I can't even leave her at church!
    d. I'm changing diapers all day—she still stools as often as she did as a newborn.

200. Which of the following reflexes is likely to have faded (integrated) in this baby?
    a. gag reflex
    b. sucking reflex
    c. extrusion reflex
    d. stepping reflex

YOUR SCORE

To self-grade your exam: Compare your answers to the Answer Key. Circle any *wrong* answers.

Total number of questions   200

Your number of *wrong* answers   _____26_____

Subtract number of wrong answers from 200   174

Total number of correct answers   _____

Multiply each correct answer by 0.5   x.05

Your Score   _____87_____

The passing grade for this exam simulation is 65%.

Congratulations if you passed!

If you did not get a score of 65 or higher, use the answer key to identify your areas of weakness, focus your study efforts in those areas, and retake the examination simulation to check your progress.

GENERAL PURPOSE - NCS® - ANSWER SHEET
SEE IMPORTANT MARKING INSTRUCTIONS ON SIDE 2

SIDE 1

GENERAL PURPOSE

NCS®

ANSWER SHEET

form no. 4521

IMPORTANT DIRECTIONS FOR MARKING ANSWERS

- Use #2 pencil only.
- Do NOT use ink or ballpoint pens.
- Make heavy black marks that fill the circle completely.
- Erase cleanly any answer you wish to change.
- Make no stray marks on the answer sheet.

EXAMPLES

WRONG
1 ① ⊗ ③ ④ ⑤

WRONG
2 ① ② ⊘ ④ ⑤

WRONG
3 ① ② ③ ◐ ⑤

RIGHT
4 ① ② ③ ● ⑤

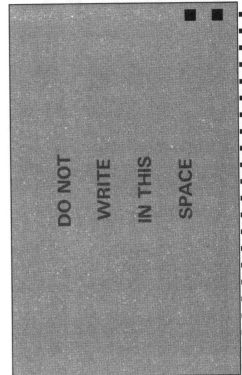

DO NOT

WRITE

IN THIS

SPACE

Trans-Optic® by NCS MPF-4521: 3231302928   Printed in U.S.A.   © 1977 by National Computer Systems, Inc.

EXAM C

1. A woman who received intravenous magnesium sulfate during labor to control her blood pressure is having trouble initiating breastfeeding. The MOST LIKELY explanation for this is:
   a. This medication can cause maternal lethargy, confusion, and muscle relaxation.
   b. The medication affected the baby's ability to suck.
   c. Her milk tastes unpleasant because of the medication.
   d. The drug reduced the amount of colostrum available, and the baby is frustrated.

2. A breastfeeding mother asks about taking an herbal remedy for migraine headaches. Your BEST response is:
   a. Herbs do not pass into milk, so whatever you take should be safe.
   b. Comfrey is a good choice.
   c. Please discuss this with your physician and a qualified herbalist.
   d. Migraines are best treated with prescription drugs.

3. A student in your prenatal class asks about the impact of labor pain-relieving medications on the baby. Your responses should include all of the following EXCEPT:
   a. Narcotic analgesics can depress the baby's breathing and sucking.
   b. Epidural anesthesia has no effect on the baby.
   c. The effect of labor drugs on the baby is dose-related.
   d. Tranquilizers potentiate the action of other drugs.

4. What is the average percent of a drug administered to a lactating woman that actually gets to the breastfeeding baby?
   a. 0.01%
   b. 0.1%
   c. 1.0%
   d. 10%

5. When would a drug given to the mother MOST readily pass into the milk?
   a. when the baby is premature
   b. in the first 4 days postbirth
   c. when the mother has a breast infection
   d. when the drug is given transdermally

6. Which drug taken by a breastfeeding mother is MOST LIKELY to have an affect on her baby?
   a. insulin
   b. digoxin
   c. caffeine
   d. warfarin

7. A pregnant mother has heard that letting epidural anesthesia wear off prior to delivery will avoid anesthesia-related breastfeeding problems. You should tell her all of the following EXCEPT:
   a. Drugs can take much longer to clear the baby's system, so there is still possible breastfeeding risk with this approach.
   b. The combination of drugs used in epidural anesthesia makes it difficult to determine which medications cause breastfeeding problems.
   c. Epidural anesthesia has minimal or no effect on the baby regardless of how long before delivery it is administered.
   d. Epidural anesthesia increases the likelihood of other birth interventions that can affect breastfeeding.

8. A breastfeeding mother must receive a radioactive isotope for diagnostic testing. How long should she wait before breastfeeding her baby again?
   a. 5 days
   b. 48 hours
   c. 5 half-lives
   d. she must completely wean

9. A mother has been having migraine headaches and asks about various remedies and their effect on her nursing 3-week-old. The remedy LEAST LIKELY to affect her baby is:
   a. acetaminophen.
   b. an herbal preparation.
   c. a homeopathic remedy.
   d. a caffeinated beverage.

10. A mother of a 2-week-old baby states that her baby's suck feels weak compared with her first baby's suck. This second baby, she states, "always seems hungry" and has also lost weight since birth. The LEAST LIKELY cause of this breastfeeding problem is:
    a. this baby is a low birthweight infant.
    b. this baby is lazy.
    c. this baby has low intraoral tone.
    d. this baby is shallowly attached at breast.

11. A healthy, fullterm newborn is found to have a total bilirubin level of 14.2 mg/dL (245 µmol/L) on the fourth day of life. The BEST recommendation is:
    a. Breastfeed the baby at least 10 times a day.
    b. Feed artificial baby milk after breastfeedings.
    c. Feed artificial baby milk for 24 hours; maintain supply through pumping.
    d. Tell the mother that this level of bilirubin is rarely a problem.

12. Which of the following approaches will be MOST helpful to assisting a breastfeeding mother who has a hearing impairment?
    a. Speak to her more slowly.
    b. Speak directly to her intepreter.
    c. Make frequent eye contact with her.
    d. Help her observe the baby's visual cues.

13. A mother reports seeing a greenish discharge come from her nipple during a bath. The MOST LIKELY cause of this discharge is:
    a. intraductal papilloma.
    b. breast abscess.
    c. infected Montgomery tubercle.
    d. mammary duct ectasia.

14. A breastfeeding mother with insulin-dependent diabetes mellitus (IDDM) is at increased risk for which of the following conditions?
    a. insufficient milk supply
    b. mastitis
    c. oversupply
    d. plugged milk ducts

15. Lactoferrin in mother's milk is beneficial to the baby because it:
    a. binds iron needed by pathogens in baby's gut.
    b. attacks and kills pathogenic bacteria in the baby's gut.
    c. promotes the absorption of lactose.
    d. provides nutrients for *Lactobacillus bifidus* in the gut.

16. A mother 5 days postbirth complains of a firm, tender area in her right breast that has persisted for 3 days, despite application of cool cabbage compresses, ice packs, and frequent milk expression using a hospital-grade electric breastpump. Your NEXT action should be:
    a. Suggest she continue this strategy for another 48 hours.
    b. Switch to warm compresses before pumping.
    c. Ask for a more thorough medical evaluation by a breast specialist.
    d. Apply a breast binder and ask her to restrict fluids.

17. Within the first minute or two of beginning a breastfeed, an infant gulps, coughs, and chokes, then releases the breast. This incident BEST describes:
    a. infant with decreased oral tone.
    b. hyperpituitarism.
    c. overactive milk ejection reflex.
    d. gastroesophageal reflux.

18. A mother complains that her baby "cries constantly." She has been feeding her baby on a strict schedule found in a popular "parenting" book. Your BEST response to her is:
    a. It is acceptable to limit your baby's feeds to 10 minutes per breast.
    b. You can give a pacifier to help your baby extend the time between feeds.
    c. Babies do best when there are no restrictions on length or frequency of breastfeeds.
    d. Giving water between feeds will get your baby onto a more regular feeding schedule.

19. Mothers of twins are LEAST likely to experience which of the following circumstances?
    a. premature birth
    b. cesarean birth
    c. intrauterine growth retardation
    d. insufficient milk supply

20. A cesarean birth is likely to affect breastfeeding in all of the following ways EXCEPT:
    a. increased maternal pain.
    b. need for maternal medications.
    c. delayed lactogenesis II.
    d. more separation of mother and infant.

21. You are writing a pamphlet on breastfeeding for new mothers. The BEST advice on whether to use one or both breasts is:
    a. Use only one breast per feed.
    b. Be sure to use both breasts per feed.
    c. Let the baby finish one breast before switching to the second breast.
    d. Switch breasts several times per feed.

22. Which of the following complementary family planning methods is MOST effective and compatible with breastfeeding?
    a. condoms
    b. implanted progestin
    c. combined oral contraceptives
    d. Lactation Amenorrhea Method

23. A mother calls on day 12 to rent a breastpump to increase her milk supply. She had an emergency cesarean, did not breastfeed or pump for the first 3 days, and has been pumping 3 to 4 times a day since then. She has not been able to get the baby to latch and feed effectively. Which of the following is MOST LIKELY to increase the rate of milk synthesis?
    a. Begin drinking $1/4$ cup of fenugreek tea three times a day.
    b. Thoroughly drain the breasts every 2 to 3 hours by nursing, pumping, and/or expressing.
    c. Put the baby to breast every 2 to 3 hours to stimulate the breasts, even if the baby does not feed well.
    d. Ask her physician to prescribe metaclopromide to increase prolactin.

24. A mother is concerned that she can pump an ounce of milk after her baby finishes feeding. The MOST LIKELY explanation for this is:
    a. The baby is not feeding effectively.
    b. Babies normally do not take all of the milk available at a given feeding.
    c. She has an oversupply of milk.
    d. Her baby does not like the taste of her milk.

25. The mother of a premature baby needs to express milk for her baby. She has relatively small breasts. Which expressing pattern is MOST likely to result in abundant supply?
    a. 6 times a day for 30 minutes per breast
    b. every 3 to 4 hours for 10 minutes per breast
    c. every 2 to 3 hours until the milk flow ceases
    d. every 1 to 2 hour during the day and once at night

26. All of the following developmental processes are interrupted by premature birth EXCEPT:
    a. bone mineralization.
    b. gut maturation.
    c. deposition of fat.
    d. hearing and taste.

27. For optimal breastfeeding, all of the following structures need to be positioned inside the infant's mouth EXCEPT:
    a. nipple epithelium.
    b. areola.
    c. milk duct outlets.
    d. alveoli.

28. What is thought to be the PRIMARY function of the Montgomery glands?
    a. color marker for baby to see
    b. lubricate the skin of the areola
    c. secrete antibiotic substances
    d. changes elasticity of areola skin

29. Which of the following orofacial disorders is NOT more prevalent in children who have been artificially fed?
    a. need for orthodontia
    b. weak masseter muscles
    c. speech and articulation disorders
    d. teeth grinding (bruxism) at night

30. A 3-year-old girl was hurt in an auto accident, and as part of her treatment, a chest tube was placed between her ribs below and distal to her right nipple. What is the WORST effect that this surgery might have on her ability to breastfeed?
    a. damage to the ductal structure
    b. damage to the blood vessels supplying the breast
    c. sever nerve pathways to the nipple
    d. cut blood vessels to the breast

31. During breastfeeding, where is the infant's tongue USUALLY placed?
    a. resting behind the alveolar ridge
    b. covering the alveolar ridge
    c. spread flat across the floor of the mouth
    d. extended past the lower lip

32. Gastroesophageal reflux may be caused by a defect in the infant's:
    a. esophagus.
    b. trachea.
    c. small intestine.
    d. large intestine.

33. Which breast structure contains the cells that secrete milk?
    a. lactiferous ducts
    b. lobules
    c. alveoli
    d. nipple

34. A woman had an emergency hysterectomy following delivery of her full-term baby. Which of the following statements is NOT relevant to her ability to breastfeed?
    a. She may have difficulty establishing full milk supply if she had excessive blood loss.
    b. She will be unable to produce milk if her ovaries were removed along with her uterus.
    c. The baby may nurse poorly due to the effect of the anesthetics used.
    d. The baby's first breastfeeding may be delayed for several hours.

35. During a difficult birth, a baby suffered damage to the hypoglossal nerve. What is the MOST LIKELY effect on breastfeeding?
    a. unable to maintain latch at breast
    b. unable to move tongue to compress breast
    c. unable to swallow
    d. unable to grasp breast with mouth/lips

36. Where is the BEST placement for the examiner's fingers when testing a nipple-areola complex for inversion?
    a. at the base of the nipple
    b. at the edge of the areola
    c. 3 inches back from the nipple tip
    d. on the nipple itself, touching the nipple base

37. A mother in your practice is rapidly becoming ill with influenza. She asks if she should continue breastfeeding her 5-month-old, exclusively breastfed child. Your responses should include all of the following EXCEPT:
    a. YES, because your milk will quickly contain specific antibodies to lessen the chance that your child will get this infection.
    b. YES, because your milk contains white cells that will help your baby fight this infection, if he gets it at all.
    c. YES, because lactation speeds up your own production of antibodies so you won't get as sick.
    d. YES, because you will get well quicker if you don't have the additional burden of preparing artificial feeds.

38. A 3-week-old exclusively breastfed baby with a strong family history of allergy has a severe reaction the first time he is fed with a cow's milk–based formula. The LEAST LIKELY explanation for this is:
    a. the baby was sensitized by intact cow milk protein that passed into mother's milk.
    b. the baby was given a bottle of formula in the hospital nursery.
    c. the mother consumed large amounts of dairy products during pregnancy.
    d. the allergic reaction was more likely due to the latex in the bottle nipple than the cow's milk.

39. All of the following conditions have been shown to be more common in people who were artificially fed as infants EXCEPT:
    a. multiple sclerosis.
    b. insulin-dependent diabetes mellitis.
    c. coronary heart disease.
    d. childhood cancers.

40. Research has identified artificial feeding as a risk factor in suboptimal neurological development, as manifested in all of the following EXCEPT:
    a. gross muscle coordination.
    b. Cognitive development (IQ).
    c. visual acuity.
    d. reading and school performance.

41. All of the following components of human milk provide antiinflammatory properties EXCEPT:
    a. complement.
    b. prostaglandins.
    c. lactoferrin.
    d. secretory IgA.

42. Which of the following is NOT an example of mutual interdependency during breastfeeding?
    a. Baby's gut closure occurs around the time he is ready for solid foods.
    b. Mother's milk contains environmental chemicals, triggering baby's immune system.
    c. Skin contact during breastfeeding helps regulate baby's temperature.
    d. Sucking at breast triggers release of gut hormones in mother and baby.

43. Breastfeeding protects the infant from allergy by all of the following methods EXCEPT:
    a. limiting the baby's exposure to nonhuman proteins.
    b. slowing or preventing the absorption of allergens through the baby's gut.
    c. protecting the baby's gut from inflammation, which weakens the mucosal barrier.
    d. providing white cells in milk, which attack the allergens directly.

44. An important consequence of adding fortifiers to human milk given to premature babies is:
    a. better long-term bone mineralization.
    b. increased risk of allergic reaction from bovine protein in fortifiers.
    c. fortifiers increase iron transport in preterm babies.
    d. fortifiers have no effect on gut transit time.

45. Soluble components of human milk that have immunologic significance include all of the following EXCEPT:
    a. interferon.
    b. fibronectin.
    c. estrogen.
    d. lactoferrin.

46. The composition of human milk varies in all of the following ways EXCEPT:
    a. fat levels vary within a feed.
    b. zinc levels decrease over time.
    c. lactose levels vary by time of day.
    d. vitamin K is highest in colostrum, then decreases.

47. Fat levels in mother's milk are highest when:
    a. the milk ejection reflex is strong.
    b. during the night.
    c. the mother eats a high-fat diet.
    d. the breast is relatively empty.

48. The ease with which human milk fat is digested by the infant is explained by all of the following EXCEPT:
    a. unsaturated fats comprise 57% of total lipids.
    b. lipases are present in the milk.
    c. lipids are encased in membranes (globules).
    d. cholesterol is the predominant lipid in human milk.

49. A breastfeeding mother who follows a strict vegetarian diet (no animal protein whatsoever) should take a supplement containing which of the following vitamins?
    a. vitamin A
    b. vitamin B6
    c. vitamin C
    d. vitamin K

50. A breastfeeding mother needs to be sure that her diet includes:
    a. additional B vitamins.
    b. plenty of liquids to ensure sufficient milk volume.
    c. an extra 1000 calories per day.
    d. her normal intake of food and drink.

51. Which of the following statements BEST describes the difference in fat content of colostrum vs. mature milk?
    a. Colostrum has 4 to 5 g/100 ml, mature milk has 2 to 3 g/100 ml of fat.
    b. Colostrum has 2 to 3 g/100 ml, mature milk has 4 to 5 g/100 ml of fat.
    c. Colostrum has roughly one quarter of the fat content of mature milk.
    d. Colostrum has 10 ml of fat and mature milk has 20 ml of fat.

52. If a mother cannot provide her milk to her baby, the World Health Organization recommends that the NEXT BEST food for her baby is:
    a. soy-based formula.
    b. cow milk–based formula.
    c. banked donor human milk.
    d. milk of another mother.

53. Research has shown that babies who received human milk have higher scores in cognitive development and vision. Which of the following milk components is MOST LIKELY to explain this difference?
    a. long-chain fatty acids
    b. short-chain fatty acids
    c. phospholipids
    d. sterols

54. Anemia in the exclusively breastfed baby is rare, because of the bioavailability of which trace element found in human milk?
    a. manganese
    b. fluoride
    c. iodine
    d. iron

55. A mother is hesitant to breastfeed because she has heard that she needs to eat a high-calorie, nutrient-rich diet during lactation. Your BEST response is:
    a. Women living under a wide variety of circumstances are capable of fully nourishing their infants by breastfeeding.
    b. Refer her to a supplemental food program to assure adequate nutrient intake.
    c. Provide her with a multivitamin-and-mineral supplement.
    d. Discourage her from breastfeeding, as her current circumstances make it doubtful that she is eating adequately.

56. The benefits of human donor milk remain similar to those of real-time breastfeeding, EXCEPT:
    a. species specific
    b. allergy prevention
    c. bioavailability
    d. HIV prevention

57. Which of the following components of human milk protects the baby by binding nutrients needed by pathogens in the baby's gut?
    a. lactoferrin
    b. lysozyme
    c. mucins
    d. oligosaccharides

58. How much milk does a newborn obtain at breast each day during the first week if breastfeeding is not restricted?
    a. 3 to 4 ounces (90 to 120 ml) per day of colostrum
    b. Increasing amounts each day as milk volume increases
    c. Less than needed for adequate hydration until day 5
    d. 25 ounces (750 ml) per day from day 2 onward

59. Giving iron-rich foods to the infant under 6 months may increase infection because:
    a. lactoferrin is bound in solution by added foods.
    b. the foods may be contaminated with pathogens.
    c. the iron-binding function of lactoferrin is overwhelmed.
    d. iron makes the infant gut more permeable to pathogens.

60. All of the following are properties of lysozmye EXCEPT:
    a. destroys *E. coli* and other bacteria
    b. increases in milk after 6 months lactation
    c. destroyed by pasteurization
    d. active against inflammation

61. A breastfeeding mother should be counseled to:
    a. drink a large glass of water whenever she breastfeeds.
    b. avoid spicy or gas-producing foods.
    c. increase her caloric intake to make enough milk.
    d. follow her usual dietary practices.

62. Pacifier (dummy, soother) use is associated with all of the following EXCEPT:
    a. improved dental development.
    b. increase in ear infections.
    c. increase in oral thrush.
    d. shorter duration of breastfeeding.

63. An effective breastpump should have all of the following features EXCEPT:
    a. transfers milk effectively
    b. painless for mother
    c. 20 to 40 cycles per minute
    d. 100 to 250 mm Hg pressure

64. Risks of using nipple shields may include all of the following EXCEPT:
    a. reduction of milk flow.
    b. changes in baby's oral-motor response.
    c. reduced prolactin levels.
    d. shortened duration of breastfeeding.

65. A mother is collecting milk for her ill, premature baby. The BEST container for her milk is:
    a. open plastic cups or bottles.
    b. soft plastic polyethylene ("nurser") bags.
    c. large containers holding several feeds.
    d. glass containers with airtight lids.

66. Which is the LEAST SIGNIFICANT risk of using a nipple shield?
    a. Reduction of milk flow.
    b. Changes in baby's oral-motor response.
    c. Difficult to keep clean.
    d. Shortened duration of breastfeeding.

67. A mother is 3 days postbirth and is worried that her milk is not flowing out, even though her breasts feel very full. She pumps 5 ml from one breast and 10 ml from the other. Your FIRST action should be:
    a. Provide her with oxytocin nasal spray.
    b. Perform alternate breast massage.
    c. Apply cold packs to her breasts.
    d. Apply hot compresses to her breasts.

68. An 18-hour-old baby has not yet successfully breastfed. He cues to feed, but cannot stay on breast. In order to help him suck better, you might advise the mother to do any of the following EXCEPT:
    a. finger-feed him to help organize his suck.
    b. cup-feed him to increase calorie intake.
    c. use a nipple shield to increase sensation to his palate.
    d. use a supplementer at breast so his suck increases milk volume.

69. A mother calls you complaining of breast pain. Her breasts are hot, hard, "knotty," and painful to the touch. She is 3 days postpartum. The FIRST suggestion you should give her is:
    a. Don't worry, your breasts will feel better in 24 hours.
    b. Use a nipple shield during feedings.
    c. Express or pump at least every 2 to 3 hours if baby can't nurse well.
    d. Restrict your fluid intake.

70. An 18-hour-old infant breastfed successfully in the first hour. Since then, he has not fed. The baby is healthy and full term and is not showing any signs of hypoglycemia. To help this baby begin breastfeeding, your FIRST action should be to have the mother:
    a. start using a nursing supplementer at breast.
    b. use a nipple shield.
    c. keep her baby skin-to-skin for the next 3 hours.
    d. give 2 ounces of formula, then try breastfeeding again.

71. A baby begins sucking on his fists about 45 minutes after the last feed ended. His mother should:
    a. give the baby a pacifier.
    b. nurse the baby again.
    c. change the baby's diaper.
    d. wait till he cries, then feed him.

72. Bacterial counts in human milk, expressed 1 hour ago, are MOST likely to be:
    a. lower, because the milk is being held at a lower temperature.
    b. lower, because macrophages in the milk are actively phagocytic.
    c. higher, because antibacterial properties of human milk work best at body temperature.
    d. higher, because human milk is a rich medium for bacterial growth.

73. Exclusive breastfeeding means that:
    a. mother's milk is transferred directly from her breast to her infant's mouth.
    b. baby receives only his mother's milk, either directly or from devices when mother is away.
    c. baby receives less than 2 oz (60 ml) of other fluids per day.
    d. baby receives no formula or solid foods.

74. Which research study design is considered to be the most rigorous?
    a. case-control
    b. randomized controlled trial
    c. quasiexperimental
    d. observational

75. Which statement describes a false negative (type II) error in a breastfeeding research study?
    a. deciding there is a difference between groups when there is no real difference
    b. deciding there is no difference between groups when there is a real difference
    c. failure to include a control group
    d. using too small a sample size to detect differences between groups

76. A research report indicates that a sample of breastfed infants had no differences in illness rates than a comparable sample of artificially fed infants. While reading this report, the MOST IMPORTANT point to look for is:
    a. the type of study used.
    b. operational definitions.
    c. the sample used.
    d. the review of the literature.

77. All of the following activities would be appropriate for celebrating World Breastfeeding Week EXCEPT:
    a. setting up a display showing environmental hazards associated with formula manufacturing.
    b. instituting a hospital policy that all mothers must breastfeed their babies at least once before the hospital staff will assist them with formula feeding.
    c. publishing a directory of local lactation support services in the community.
    d. printing "Breastfeeding Welcome Here" stickers/signs for local businesses and employers.

78. Which of the following activities is NOT prohibited by the International Code of Marketing of Breast-Milk Substitutes?
    a. giving "gift packs" containing samples and coupons for formula to new mothers at hospital discharge
    b. providing detailed information on product composition to health workers
    c. advertising toddler formula on local television stations
    d. showing a picture of a happy baby on the label of infant formula containers

79. Compared with milk from mothers who deliver at term, milk from mothers who deliver preterm is:
    a. higher in lactose, vitamins, and minerals.
    b. higher in protein, sodium, and chloride.
    c. lower in calcium, magnesium, and phosphorus.
    d. equivalent in immunologic properties.

80. The management of mother-baby couples addressed in the WHO/UNICEF Baby Friendly Hospital Initiative (Ten Steps to Successful Breastfeeding) applies to:
    a. all babies, no matter how fed.
    b. all artificially fed babies.
    c. all breastfed babies.
    d. breastfed babies who room-in.

81. Breastfeeding is a core strategy of child survival programs because it provides all of the following health advantages EXCEPT:
    a. baby's first immunization.
    b. best nutrition for first 12 months.
    c. lower rates of infant mortality.
    d. long-term reduction in diabetes risk.

82. According to the WHO/UNICEF "Ten Steps to Successful Breast-feeding," a mother should:
    a. remain in the hospital with her baby for 48 hours after delivery.
    b. be given a breast pump.
    c. breastfeed her baby within a half-hour of birth.
    d. be informed about the risks of feeding infant formula.

83. A mother is divorcing the father of her 7-month-old breastfeeding child. The father wants her to wean immediately so the child will not miss his mother in the middle of the night. The LC has been asked by the mother to testify as an expert witness. The LC's role would include all of the following actions EXCEPT:
    a. charging your usual fees for this service.
    b. preparing a written statement.
    c. giving your professional opinion about the baby's needs.
    d. encouraging the mother to comply with the father's wishes.

84. Your client's baby is having problems breastfeeding and appears to have oral thrush. She requests that you NOT report your findings to the baby's pediatrician. Your BEST response is to:
    a. Inform her that lactation consultants are required to communicate relevant information to the primary health care provider(s).
    b. Agree to keep this information confidential.
    c. Provide information on over-the-counter treatments for oral thrush.
    d. Immediately discontinue providing breastfeeding care to this mother.

85. When doing a review of the literature for a research study, which sources are MOST IMPORTANT to include?
    a. review articles, which analyze several studies
    b. textbooks that explain basic concepts
    c. peer-reviewed journal report of research, written by the researcher
    d. lectures given at large conferences by well-known speakers

86. You are about to assess a breastfeeding mother and her baby. What should you do FIRST?
    a. obtain written consent from the mother
    b. weigh the baby
    c. examine the mother's breasts
    d. wash your hands

87. Which of the following behaviors suggests that the woman has NOT moved through normal developmental tasks of pregnancy?
    a.   wearing maternity clothing in her second trimester
    b.   choosing possible baby names
    c.   giving up smoking
    d.   waiting until the third trimester to tell family members of her pregnancy

88. Accessory nipple or breast tissue may be found in any of the following locations EXCEPT:
    a.   axilla.
    b.   inguinal region.
    c.   near the umbilicus.
    d.   outer thigh.

89. Separating mothers and babies shortly after birth has all of the following consequences EXCEPT:
    a.   increased rates of infection
    b.   improved rest for mother
    c.   increase in infant stress hormones
    d.   difficulty initiating breastfeeding

90. A mother is planning to go back to work after her baby is born. You can best support her breastfeeding by encouraging her to do all of the following strategies EXCEPT:
    a.   use the maximum amount of maternity leave to which she is entitled.
    b.   discuss part-time or flexible schedules with her supervisor.
    c.   plan to bottle-feed with formula while at work and continue breastfeeding during off-duty hours.
    d.   investigate child care at her work site or nearby.

91. "External gestation" includes all of the following behaviors EXCEPT:
    a.   baby sleeps through the night in his own room.
    b.   mother carries baby in a sling or tie-on carrier many hours a day.
    c.   frequent breastfeeding around the clock.
    d.   mother takes baby to work with her.

92. Of the following options for mothers returning to work, which is the LEAST likely to protect the breastfeeding relationship?
    a.   on-site child care
    b.   extended paid maternity leave
    c.   flexible working hours
    d.   facilities for collecting and storing milk

93. A mother's psychological and emotional reaction to birth is LEAST LIKELY to be affected by:
    a.) the mother's age
    b. whether this pregnancy was planned
    c. how her spouse/partner reacted to the pregnancy
    d. temperament and health of her baby

94. A health care provider wants to encourage pregnant woman to choose breastfeeding. Which statement is MOST supportive of breastfeeding?
    a. Are you considering breastfeeding?
    b.) What have you heard about breastfeeding?
    c. Are you going to breastfeed or bottlefeed?
    d. You aren't thinking about breastfeeding, are you?

95. Breastfeeding care in the modern industrialized health care system is impeded MOST by its:
    a. heightened emphasis on the baby at the expense of the mother.
    b. heightened emphasis on the mother at the expense of the baby.
    c.) failure to consider the breastfeeding dyad as a unique biological unit.
    d. failure to consider the role of the father in solving breastfeeding problems.

96. A birth plan designed to optimize breastfeeding success should include all of the following EXCEPT:
    a. place of birth where mother feels safest.
    b. continuous support by a labor companion.
    c. freedom to move and adopt an upright posture.
    d.) medications for pain relief available early in labor.

97. According to studies of breastfed babies in an industrialized society, which of the following feeding patterns most closely approximates that of an exclusively breastfed 3-month-old baby?
    a. 4 to 6 feeds per day, total 60 minutes or more
    b. 6 to 8 feeds per day, total 100 minutes or more
    c. 8 to 10 feeds per day, total 120 minutes or more
    d.) 10 to 12 feeds per day, total 140 minutes or more

98. Benefits to mother and baby of breastfeeding past 12 months include all of the following EXCEPT:
    a.) continued source of most calories in baby's diet.
    b. continued immune protection of baby.
    c. mutual pleasure in the relationship.
    d. reassurance of mother's permanence.

99. A mother asks about a book she has read, which recommends letting a baby "cry it out" to teach him to sleep all night by 3 months of age. The authors claim that responding immediately to baby's cries will teach the baby to be manipulative. Based on Erickson and Piaget's work regarding the development of trust, your BEST response to her is:

    a. Three-month-old babies are learning trust. Your NOT responding to him teaches him that he can't trust you.
    b. The book is correct. Babies can learn to self-soothe at that age.
    c. Babies learn to manipulate parents at an early age. You can learn to differentiate his cries of real distress.
    d. By 3 months, his ability to trust you is already developed, and crying it out won't hurt him.

100. A nursing strike by a 7- to 9-month-old child is likely to be precipitated by any of the following EXCEPT:

    a. illness in the infant.
    b. mother's reaction to baby biting during feeds.
    c. change in mother's soap, perfume, or deodorant.
    d. infant's readiness to wean.

101. What window (age) period most likely represents the biologic normal end of breastfeeding for human infants?

    a. 9 to 15 months
    b. around 18 months
    c. around 24 months
    d. $2\frac{1}{2}$ to 7 years

102. A mother wants to continue breastfeeding her 18-month-old child during a subsequent pregnancy. A neighbor told her to wean so that the toddler's breastfeeding does not trigger premature labor. Your BEST response is:

    a. Suggest she immediately wean the older baby.
    b. Tell her breastfeeding during a normal pregnancy is not harmful to either child.
    c. Suggest she use lanolin to prevent nipple pain during the pregnancy.
    d. Recommend that she discontinue sexual relations so that uterine contractions do not jeopardize the pregnancy.

103. A mother is concerned about her baby's feeding pattern. The baby nurses 10 to 30 minutes on one breast, then self-detaches. Your BEST response to her is:
    a. This is a normal, common pattern.
    b. Babies get all they need in the first 10 minutes.
    c. Your baby has a sucking problem.
    d. Your let-down reflex is too slow.

104. A mother asks you when her baby will likely wean from breastfeeding. Your BEST response is:
    a. She should wean at 12 months to prevent dental decay.
    b. Continue to breastfeed at least 24 months and as long as you and your baby desire.
    c. Your baby will begin weaning at 6 months and complete weaning by 1 year.
    d. He'll probably want to continue exclusive breastfeeding until 12 months, then begin weaning.

105. In order to breastfeed successfully, it is MOST important for a mother of twins to:
    a. get at least 6 straight hours of sleep each night.
    b. learn to feed her babies simultaneously.
    c. use a nursing pillow.
    d. follow her babies' cues.

106. Epidural narcotic or anesthetic drugs given to the laboring woman may have all of the following effects EXCEPT:
    a. improved neonatal neuromuscular coordination.
    b. longer second stage of labor.
    c. increased risk of cesarean birth.
    d. increased risk for forceps or vacuum-assisted birth.

107. All of the following structures are found in fetal circulation EXCEPT:
    a. ductus venosus.
    b. foramen ovale.
    c. ductus arteriosus.
    d. foramen magnum.

108. The normal and safest nighttime sleep and breastfeeding pattern for the 3-month-old, exclusively breastfed baby is:
    a. Mother and baby share a bed and feed several times at night.
    b. Baby sleeps in another room away from parents.
    c. Baby is put to bed at a regular time and allowed to self-comfort to go to sleep.
    d. Baby is nursed to sleep, then put down with a pacifier in a crib.

109. A full-term baby breastfeeds effectively in only one position, and only on one of his mother's breasts. The LEAST LIKELY explanation is:
    a. the baby has a broken clavicle.
    b. one side of the baby's head was injured during birth.
    c. the mother has a stronger let-down in one breast.
    d. the mother fed him in this position shortly after birth and he doesn't like change.

110. Lack of eye contact and little talking or caressing of her infant should alert you to the possibility of:
    a. neurologically impaired infant.
    b. neurologically impaired mother.
    c. developmentally delayed infant.
    d. clinically depressed mother.

111. A mother expresses fear that her milk supply is faltering. She is nursing on cue at least 12 times per 24 hours, and is feeling tired and chilly. Which is the MOST LIKELY cause of these signs?
    a. low serum prolactin levels
    b. low thyroid level
    c. anemia
    d. chronic fatigue syndrome

112. A mother is having trouble keeping her 40-hour-old son awake. Your suggestions should include all of the following EXCEPT:
    a. Try a cool cloth on his face.
    b. Flick his feet with your finger.
    c. Gently massage his back, arms and legs.
    d. Place him on your chest skin-to-skin.

113. A mother is planning for surgery to repair her 5-month-old child's cleft palate. Your suggestions would include all of the following EXCEPT:
    a. Wean your baby at least a week before the surgery.
    b. Prepare to stay with your baby around the clock.
    c. Practice expressing milk in case the baby cannot nurse directly.
    d. Expect your baby to nurse very frequently afterward for awhile.

114. A newborn baby, 6 hours old, is awake and alert but having trouble breastfeeding. Which of the following is the LEAST likely cause of his difficulty?

    a. Mother received antibiotic treatment for group B streptococcus during labor.
    b. Mother was given epidural anesthesia 4 hours before delivery.
    c. Mother received narcotic analgesia immediately prior to delivery.
    d. Mother's labor was stimulated by pitocin.

115. When revising or creating policies relating to breastfeeding, which of the following provides the WEAKEST evidence for the policy?

    a. systematic reviews and metaanalyses
    b. randomized controlled trials
    c. cross-sectional surveys
    d. case reports

116. A 10-hour-old healthy, full-term baby has a blood sugar level of 36 mg/dL (2 mmol/L). The BEST treatment is to:

    a. ask the mother to breastfeed her baby.
    b. do nothing.
    c. give the baby a bottle of glucose water.
    d. give the baby 30 ml (1 oz) of artificial baby milk.

117. Women who do not breastfeed their babies are at higher risk for all of the following conditions related to reproduction EXCEPT:

    a. postpartum hemorrhage.
    b. delayed return to prepregnancy weight.
    c. menstrual irregularities and pain.
    d. closely spaced pregnancies.

118. Which of the following practices is an appropriate precaution to take in the hospital labor and delivery (birthing) area?

    a. Make sure the baby can take formula by bottle before attempting to breastfeed.
    b. Read the hospital policies to the mother before she is admitted in labor.
    c. Deep suction the baby before feeding with oral fluids including breastmilk or colostrum.
    d. Give the baby only mother's own milk or colostrum unless medically indicated.

119. A woman with a 5-month-old exclusively breastfed baby is prescribed Amoxicillin for her breast infection. The possible consequences for the infant are:
    a. interference with bilirubin binding.
    b. vomiting and dehydration.
    c. none.
    d. diarrhea or loose stools.

120. Which category of drugs is LEAST LIKELY to remain in breastmilk after the mother stops taking the drug?
    a. marijuana
    b. cocaine
    c. amphetamines
    d. alcohol

121. A mother complains of sudden-onset sore nipple when her baby is 10 months old. To identify the cause, you would ask all of the following questions EXCEPT:
    a. Did you recently begin taking birth control pills?
    b. Is your baby taking any solid foods or artificial baby milk?
    c. Have you or your baby taken an antibiotic recently?
    d. Has anyone in the family been sick with an infection?

122. Which of the following behaviors is LEAST LIKELY to occur in the breastfeeding child of this age?
    a. Mother and child have a "code word" for breastfeeding.
    b. Child can postpone nursing for short periods.
    c. Nighttime breastfeeding increases child's risk of dental caries.
    d. Child receives substantial immune protection from breastfeeding.

123. This mother of a 3-month-old began feeling pinpoint pain on her nipple tip 2 days ago. The pain is MOST LIKELY due to a:
    a. plugged duct.
    b. plugged nipple pore.
    c. bacterial infection.
    d. sucking blister.

124. This mother's baby is 8 days old. The MOST LIKELY cause of the condition pictured is:
    a. normal breastfeeding.
    b. baby is tongue-tied.
    c. baby is not latching deeply.
    d. baby is biting during feeds.

125. The bulge on this mother's breast is MOST LIKELY:
     a. a plugged duct.
     (b.) a galactocele.
     c. mastitis.
     d. an abscess.

126. After assessing this baby, your FIRST SUGGESTION to the mother should be:
     a. Use a nipple shield during feeds.
     b. Your baby needs an oral surgery consult immediately.
     c. Let's see how your baby does at breast.
     d. Pump your milk and feed with a bottle today.

127. This 8-day-old infant has been at breast constantly since birth. His mother complains of nipple pain and states that her baby makes a clicking sound, and loses his grasp of her nipple frequently during the feed. You have corrected her latch-on technique. Your NEXT action should be:
     a. Provide her with a sterile nipple shield.
     b. Instruct her to use several different breastfeeding positions.
     c. Instruct her in suck training to correct the baby's sucking.
     (d.) Refer her to a health professional qualified to perform a frenotomy.

128. This condition is MOST LIKELY associated with which of the following?
     a. delayed or inadequate treatment of mastitis
     b. ductal yeast infection
     c. transmission of oral bacteria from the baby's mouth
     d. bruising or trauma to the breast

129. What is the MOST LIKELY situation leading to this breast condition?
     a. The child is over a year and using the mother's breast as a pacifier.
     b. The mother did not wash her breasts after each nursing.
     c. The child is biting during breastfeeding.
     (d.) The child has an oral infection that was transmitted to the nipple skin.

130. What is the LEAST LIKELY cause of the condition shown?
     a. Paget's disease
     b. plugged nipple pore
     c. persistent wound from baby's tongue thrust
     d. nipple thrust (candida)

131. You would recommend this technique for all of the following EXCEPT:
    a. premature baby
    b. separation of mother and baby for any reason
    c. mother taking a contraindicated medication
    d. mother has a history of sexual abuse

132. This mother's nipple pain has persisted for over 2 weeks. You would check her baby for all of the following conditions EXCEPT:
    a. micrognathia.
    b. short lingual frenulum.
    c. tongue thrust movements.
    d. cleft of the soft palate.

133. This baby prefers this position and has significant difficulty nursing in other positions. What is the MOST LIKELY cause of this preference?
    a. interesting objects on one side of his crib
    b. mother feeds only on one breast
    c. torticollis
    d. ankyloglossia

134. The mother of this infant is MOST LIKELY to complain of:
    a. difficulty getting baby to latch on.
    b. itching, burning nipples.
    c. vaginal discharge.
    d. plugged ducts.

135. This mother is 4 days postpartum. All of the following recommendations are appropriate EXCEPT:
    a. Apply cool cabbage compresses to the lump in your right armpit.
    b. Feed your baby at least every 2 to 3 hours or more often if he cues.
    c. Apply hot compresses to help milk flow in your left breast.
    d. Use cool compresses after feeds if breasts feel full.

136. This breastfeeding child lives in a northern latitude. To prevent rickets, you would recommend all of the following EXCEPT:
    a. Expose the child's face to sunlight for 20 minutes every day.
    b. Mother should take a vitamin D supplement.
    c. Mother should expose her face and head to sunlight for 2 hours a week.
    d. Give the child a vitamin D supplement regardless of symptoms.

137. This child has recently begun solid foods. Based on the condition pictured, she is likely to also have any of the other reactions listed below EXCEPT:
    a. wheezing.
    b. colic.
    c. sleepiness.
    d. irritability.

138. This baby's behavior as shown is MOST LIKELY to be caused by:
    a. overfeeding at breast.
    b. too-vigorous burping after feeds.
    c. allergy to something in mother's diet.
    d. gastroesophageal reflux.

139. The mother of this baby is practicing the Lactation Amenorrhea Method of family planning. Which behavior would NOT diminish the effectiveness of the method?
    a. intercourse more than twice a week.
    b. relief bottle every other day.
    c. baby sleeping through the night
    d. return of menstruation

140. This baby feeds for 30 to 45 minutes at each breast, each feeding, in the exact position shown in this picture. The MOST LIKELY cause of this behavior is:
    a. normal behavior
    b. disorganized sucking
    c. mother has low milk supply
    d. delayed clearing of labor drugs

141. What is the MOST LIKELY conclusion you could draw from the appearance of this lactating woman's breasts?
    a. The smaller breast has insufficient glandular tissue.
    b. The larger breast is making much more milk than the smaller.
    c. The baby most recently nursed on the smaller breast.
    d. Lactation and breastfeeding are proceeding smoothly for her and her baby.

142. What is the MOST LIKELY age of this baby?
    a. 36 weeks gestational age
    b. 38 weeks gestational age
    c. 2 days postbirth
    d. 4 days postbirth

143. All of the following will improve this mother's breastfeeding success EXCEPT:
    a. wearing breast shells several hours a day for the remainder of her pregnancy.
    b. learning nonpharmaceutical methods of pain relief for labor.
    c. vigorously pulling and stretching her nipples several times a day.
    d. arranging for 24-hour rooming-in starting at birth.

144. The condition pictured appeared suddenly 3 days postbirth. The FIRST suggestion you would give to this mother is:
    a. Try massaging the plug of milk toward your nipple.
    b. See whether the lump changes size after you nurse your baby.
    c. Put hot compresses on the swollen area.
    d. Make an appointment with a breast surgeon for a biopsy.

145. When would this mother's baby get milk with the highest fat content?
    a. the last 5 minutes of each feed on either breast
    b. after nursing several times on one breast
    c. in the middle of the night
    d. when mother is eating a high-fat diet

146. This mother asked for advice on family planning. She wishes to continue breastfeeding yet does not want to become pregnant again. Your BEST response to her is:
    a. Begin taking a progestin-only oral contraceptive.
    b. Use a condom every time you have intercourse.
    c. An intrauterine devise is your best option.
    d. Breastfeed exclusively around the clock without supplements or pacifiers.

147. What is this mother doing with the hand that is not holding the device?
    a. tapping the breast to aid milk let-down
    b. massaging milk toward the nipple to increase collected volume
    c. pressing her breast more deeply into the flange
    d. stroking the skin surface to increase milk synthesis

148. The rash on this baby's face appeared when he began receiving supplements of cow's milk–based artificial baby milk. What is the MOST LIKELY cause of the rash?
    a. normal infant acne
    b. reaction to nonhuman protein in the artificial baby milk
    c. presence of bovine antigen in mother's milk
    d. allergic reaction to latex in bottle teat

149. What is the MOST LIKELY reason this baby cannot make a good seal on the mother's breast?
    a. The tongue is trough-shaped.
    b. The tongue is too thick.
    c. The baby has a small mouth opening.
    d. The lingual frenulum is short and tight.

150. This baby's mother complains of clicking and smacking during breastfeeds. The MOST LIKELY explanation is:
    a. high-domed palate prevents deep latch.
    b. tongue-tie prevents deep attachment.
    c. tongue shape causes intermittent loss of seal.
    d. buccal fat pads are interfering with tongue movement.

151. This mother's baby was tongue-tied and was having trouble latching on and breastfeeding. The MOST LIKELY maternal reason for the baby's difficulty is:
    a. her nipple is somewhat short and flat.
    b. her breast is engorged, preventing deep latch.
    c. her nipple is very small, and the baby couldn't feel it.
    d. her nipple is very large, and the baby was choking on it.

152. The baby's tongue was pressing this mother's nipple against the baby's hard palate. Which cranial nerve was MOST responsible for this tongue movement?
    a. spinal accessory
    b. vagus
    c. hypoglossal
    d. trigeminal

153. The lumps on this woman's areola are MOST LIKELY due to which of the following?
    a. irritation from wet bra pads
    b. infected Montgomery glands
    c. poison ivy
    d. normal anatomy

154. This mother is concerned about the condition shown in this picture. Which of the following is the MOST APPROPRIATE response?
   a. You may have Reynaud's syndrome. Keep the room warm when you breastfeed.
   b. The lumps are Montgomery glands, which help lubricate the skin. They're normal.
   c. This appears to be an allergic reaction. Did you recently start wearing a new bra?
   d. May I check your baby's mouth to see if he has a thrush infection?

155. The nipple shown in this picture is:
   a. inverted.
   b. retracted.
   c. folded.
   d. flat.

156. This woman is planning to become pregnant. She is concerned about her nipple size and worried that her baby will have difficulty breastfeeding. Your BEST response to her is:
   a. Yes, your small nipple may be a problem.
   b. Small nipples work just fine—in fact, they may make breast-feeding easier
   c. Be sure to pull and roll your nipples daily throughout pregnancy
   d. Wear breast shells during your pregnancy to increase eversion

157. When a breastfeeding baby has this condition, the FIRST thing you would do is:
   a. treat the baby and mother's breast for a fungal infection.
   b. check the child for other manifestations of allergic responses.
   c. advise the mother to change the baby's diaper more frequently.
   d. have the mother apply a cortisone ointment on the rash.

158. What is the MOST LIKELY cause of the condition pictured?
   a. acidic urine from human milk feedings
   b. yeast infection (candida)
   c. allergic reaction to cow milk protein passing through mother's milk
   d. sensitivity to chemicals in disposable diapers

159. After examining this woman's breasts, you would do all of the following actions EXCEPT:
   a. instruct her on better cleaning procedures for her breastpump.
   b. provide her with a nipple shield to wear during feeds.
   c. request that the primary care provider culture the baby's mouth.
   d. recommend that she wean immediately.

160. About how much milk will this baby receive each day during the next week if breastfeeding is not restricted?
    a. The baby gets about 150 ml/day (5 oz/day) of colostrum.
    b. The baby gets increasing amounts each day as milk volume increases.
    c. The baby needs a supplement until day 5 when mom's supply is sufficient.
    d. The baby gets 750 ml/day (25 oz/day) from day 2 onward.

161. Offering this child family (complementary) foods in addition to breastmilk is appropriate at this age for all of the following reasons EXCEPT:
    a. she is about 6 months old.
    b. she is reaching for table foods.
    c. the nutritional quality of mother's milk is diminishing.
    d. she enjoys the social aspects of family mealtimes.

162. Breast shells would be MOST helpful for this mother to:
    a. evert her nipples.
    b. protect the damaged skin from clothing.
    c. protect the nipple tip from the baby's palate.
    d. reduce areolar edema.

163. The equipment shown in this picture is appropriately used for all of the following EXCEPT:
    a. inducing lactation when the baby is adopted.
    b. supplementing a neurologically impaired baby at breast.
    c. correcting a baby's dysfunctional sucking pattern.
    d. aiding the mother to reestablish breastfeeding after an interruption.

164. This mother complains of sharp nipple pain. Your suggestions should include all of the following EXCEPT:
    a. apply purified lanolin to the irritated area.
    b. wear a silicone nipple shield during feeds.
    c. wear breast shells between feeds.
    d. bring the baby deeply onto the breast.

165. This device should have all of the following features EXCEPT:
    a. can cycle 40 to 60 times per minute
    b. creates vacuum pressure in the range of 100 to 300 mm Hg
    c. flange diameter easily accommodates the mother's nipple
    d. requires sterilization after every use

166. Which is the LEAST appropriate treatment for this condition?
    a. antifungal therapy
    b. infant continues to breastfeed
    c. fit mother with a breast binder
    d. antibiotic therapy

167. This mother is worried that her left breast is larger than her right. Your FIRST response should be:
    a. the left breast appears to have mastitis.
    b. different breast sizes are very common.
    c. what size were your breasts before pregnancy?
    d. the left will clearly make more milk than the right.

168. This mother says her nipples started itching and stinging a few days ago. The MOST LIKELY cause of her symptoms is:
    a. dry skin.
    b. eczema.
    c. nipple thrush.
    d. positional soreness.

169. Which of the following suggestions is MOST LIKELY to be helpful for the condition pictured?
    a. Air-dry after feedings.
    b. Expose the breast to a sunlamp placed about 1 ft (0.3 m) away.
    c. Use moist wound healing techniques or preparations.
    d. Cover with a breast shell between feeds.

170. This baby had trouble latching and staying on breast and was not gaining weight. The mother's nipples were very painful at every feed. Attempting a deeper latch and better positioning did not improve the situation. The practitioner shown is MOST LIKELY performing which of the following procedures?
    a. frenectomy
    b. frenotomy
    c. tonsillectomy
    d. myringotomy

171. Which visual aspect of this baby's latch is LEAST LIKELY to be a problem?
    a. angle of the lips/mouth is about 90 degrees
    b. puckering along the naso-labial crease
    c. chin barely touches the breast
    d. areola is nearly completely in baby's mouth

172. This baby's mother is concerned about a clicking, smacking sound that occurs during nursing. Her nipples are mildly tender. Your FIRST intervention would be:
    a. Refer her for evaluation of the baby's tongue masculature.
    b. Assure good alignment and deep latch at breast.
    c. Perform a digital exam to assess tongue movement.
    d. Reassure her that some nipple tenderness is normal in early lactation.

173. This mother has not completed State III of her labor. Her baby is healthy. The NEXT thing you should do is:
    a. get her to a hospital.
    b. put the baby to breast.
    c. give her oxygen for her exhaustion.
    d. have her assume a supine position.

174. This mother's baby is four months old. The MOST IMPORTANT thing you would do to help relieve this mother's discomfort is:
    a. teach her how to keep her baby from squirming during feeds.
    b. assist her baby to take more of the breast during latch-on.
    c. provide a silicone nipple shield to reduce abrasion on the nipple skin.
    d. help her get treatment for a probable nipple thrush infection.

175. This condition began when the child started taking solid foods. What would your FIRST management strategy be?
    a. Discontinue all solid food until the rash clears up.
    b. Mother should stop consuming dairy products.
    c. Take a thorough history of the mother and baby's food intake.
    d. Refer the dyad to a dermatologist.

176. This mother's baby is 20 hours old and has not yet effectively latched on and breastfed. What would be your FIRST strategy to help them?
    a. Place a silicone nipple shield over her nipples during feeds.
    b. Have the mother pump her breasts to firm and evert the nipple tissue.
    c. Remove her clothing and place the baby skin-to-skin on her chest.
    d. Suggest she begin suck training to coordinate the baby's suck.

177. This mother complains of pinpoint pain at the 1:00 position on her nipple. Your FIRST suggestion to her would be:
    a. use a sterile instrument to lift the flap of skin over that pore.
    b. soak the nipple tip in warm water, then try to "pop" out the plug.
    c. coat the nipple with an antifungal preparation.
    d. nurse frequently on that side as often as the baby is willing.

178.   How would you document this baby's oral configuration?
   a.   Normal tongue position.
   b.   Tongue is bunched or humped.
   c.   The tongue stays behind the inferior alveolar ridge.
   d.   The baby has a poor tongue position.

179.   This baby feeds at least 10 times a day, including 2 to 3 feeds at night. Her grandmother has advised her mother that she should be feeding her rice cereal and strained fruits. Your BEST response to her is:
   a.   This frequency of feeding is normal for a baby of this age.
   b.   If she has been nursing this frequently for several days, then you apparently cannot make enough milk for her.
   c.   She does not need solids, but she should be sleeping through the night.
   d.   If she is 4 months old, it is good to start her on supplemental foods.

180.   This mother is 36 weeks pregnant. Your BEST recommendation would be:
   a.   rub your nipples with a towel twice a day.
   b.   be sure to breastfeed in the first hour postbirth.
   c.   pull and roll the nipple to stretch it.
   d.   you won't be able to breastfeed.

181.   What technique is being shown in this picture?
   a.   checking for cleft palate
   b.   suck training
   c.   digital oral assessment
   d.   checking for short frenulum

182.   This baby's mother complains about clicking and smacking during breastfeeds that has continued since the baby was a newborn. She has just begun taking solid food. The FIRST action you would do is:
   a.   check for a cleft of the soft palate.
   b.   observe a full breastfeeding session.
   c.   have the baby's doctor diagnose or rule out thrush infection.
   d.   ask the mother to record what foods the baby has taken in the past 24 hours.

183.   What is the FIRST thing you would recommend to increase this mother's comfort during breastfeeding?
   a.   Bring the baby further onto the breast.
   b.   Use an antifungal cream on her nipples.
   c.   Apply lanolin after nursings.
   d.   Use a different brand of bra pad.

184. Compared with the NCHS growth charts, this child gained weight faster than expected in her first three months, but now is slightly below the same percentile curve. All other development milestones are normal. Your BEST recommendation to his mother is:
    a. Continue what you are doing. His growth pattern is normal for breastfed babies.
    b. Begin feeding him more solid foods to increase his weight.
    c. Take away his chewing toys and pacifiers as they are distracting him from eating.
    d. Supplement with a cow's milk–based infant formula because he needs more calcium for growth.

185. This mother just finished pumping her milk. The MOST LIKELY explanation for the condition pictured is:
    a. nipple thrush.
    b. pump flange was too small in diameter.
    c. Reynaud's phenomenon.
    d. pump has everted her nipples.

186. This mother is likely to experience all of the following EXCEPT:
    a. mutual enjoyment of breastfeeding.
    b. sibling rivalry for the breast.
    c. babies interact with each other during feeds.
    d. higher risk of milk stasis.

187. This mother is becoming annoyed with her child's behavior during nursings, including the action shown in the photo. Your FIRST response to her should be:
    a. Well, then it's time to think about weaning him.
    b. Many children try to nurse while they play with toys.
    c. Driving his toy truck across your chest during nursing really bothers you.
    d. Grab his hand and don't let him play with your body during feeds.

188. Mother support groups are MOST effective for which of the following reasons?
    a. Groups meet in members' homes.
    b. The group leader is highly trained.
    c. Cost for support groups is usually low.
    d. Mothers hear other mothers' ideas.

189. Which is the LEAST LIKELY reason this child breastfeeds 4 to 8 times every day, including 1 to 2 times at night?
    a. Mother is pressuring the child to gratify her own desires.
    b. Child is recovering from gastroenteritis.
    c. Child is allergic to many foods.
    d. Mother is recovering from a hospital stay where child could not visit.

190. This breastfed baby's mother feels that he should learn how to sleep for at least 8 straight hours at night. Your BEST response to her is:
    a. Most babies of this age still need to breastfeed around the clock.
    b. He is too young now, but he should be sleeping through the night soon.
    c. If you don't go to him for a few nights, he will learn to sleep longer.
    d. He does not need to breastfeed at night if he weighs at least 12 lbs. (5.4 kg).

191. The age of this baby is MOST LIKELY:
    a. 4 months.
    b. 6 months.
    c. 8 months.
    d. 10 months.

192. The support being received by this mother helps foster all of the following EXCEPT:
    a. improved maternal-infant bonding.
    b. breastfeeding duration.
    c. maternal self-esteem.
    d. increased maternal dependency.

193. Common breastfeeding behaviors of babies at this age include all of the following EXCEPT:
    a. mother and baby develop "code word" for nursing.
    b. baby is taking family foods well.
    c. increased ability for baby to postpone feeds.
    d. baby passes stool during most feeds.

194. Which of the following events are NOT associated with a baby of this age?
    a. Breastfeeding is going smoothly.
    b. Baby sleeps 8 to 9 hours at night.
    c. Baby looks to locate interesting sounds.
    d. Baby recognizes mother and smiles.

195.   Which statement BEST describes the reason this baby would begin reaching for table (family) food?
   a.   The baby is developmentally ready for solid food.
   b.   The mother's milk supply is no longer adequate.
   c.   The baby is just imitating and will not be ready for family foods for some time.
   d.   The baby is jealous because everyone else is eating "real food."

196.   Which of the following is the MOST common breastfeeding behavior of a child at this age?
   a.   Biting at the end of feeds.
   b.   Nursing strike.
   c.   Easily distracted while nursing. — 4-6 months
   d.   Playfulness and vocalization during feeds. over 1 yr

197.   This baby's mother complains that her baby has increased her night feeds. Your responses should include all of the following EXCEPT:
   a.   this is normal behavior at this age.
   b.   try going to a quieter, darker place.
   c.   you can try feeding solid foods during the day.
   d.   night feeds are important to your baby at this age.

198.   The infant behavioral state shown in this picture is:
   a.   active alert.
   b.   quiet alert.
   c.   light sleep.
   d.   drowsy.

199.   This child's nursing behavior is:
   a.   highly unusual at this age.
   b.   indicative of attachment disorder.
   c.   normal for a child this age.
   d.   likely to cause dental caries.

200.   What is the LEAST LIKELY reason that a grandmother would engage in the behavior shown?
   a.   competition with the baby's mother.
   b.   soothe the baby while mother finishes a nap.
   c.   baby has a medical condition that requires upright posture.
   d.   genuine affection for her grandchild.

YOUR SCORE

To self-grade your exam: Compare your answers to the Answer Key. Circle any *wrong* answers.

Total number of questions	200
Your number of *wrong* answers	_____
Subtract number of wrong answers from 200	
Total number of correct answers	_____
Multiply each correct answer by 0.5	_____ x.05

Your Score _____

The passing grade for this exam simulation is 65%.

Congratulations if you passed!

If you did not get a score of 65 or higher, use the answer key to identify your areas of weakness, focus your study efforts in those areas, and retake the examination simulation to check your progress.

Exam Answers

EXAM A

1. The answer is D. Even though Amoxicillin is considered compatible with breastfeeding, the infant may develop diarrhea or loose stools. (Pharmacology; 4-6 months; Knowledge; Difficulty 4)

2. The answer is A. Overhydration during labor may cause breast, nipple and areolar edema, making latch-on difficult for the baby. (Pharmacology; Labor/birth (perinatal); Application; Difficulty 5)

3. The answer is D. Anti-inflammatory drugs are generally compatible with breastfeeding. The other statements are false. (Pharmacology; 15-28 days; Knowledge; Difficulty 3)

4. The answer is D. Lipid solubility facilitates transfer of drugs into mother's milk. The other factors inhibit drug transfer to milk. (Pharmacology; General Principles; Knowledge; Difficulty 4)

5. The answer is A. Determining the safety of maternal medications is reserved for appropriately licensed health care providers. The other three responses are appropriate for the lactation consultant. (Pharmacology; General Principles; Application; Difficulty 5)

6. The answer is A. The concentration of drug in the milk is nearly always proportional to the level in maternal plasma. (Pharmacology; General Principles; Knowledge; Difficulty 2)

7. The answer is A. Pain-relieving drugs work on the central nervous system and therefore are highly lipid soluble, and sequester in the infant brain. The other answers are incorrect. (Pharmacology; Labor/birth (perinatal); Application; Difficulty 3)

8. The answer is A. Antibiotic drugs have no documented affect on the fetus or newborn's ability to breastfeed. The other choices may contribute to breastfeeding difficulties. (Pharmacology; Labor/birth (perinatal); Application; Difficulty 2)

9. The answer is A. In order for a maternal medication to affect the baby, it must pass into milk and be ingested by the baby. Drugs that are not absorbed from the GI tract are very low risk because the baby's GI tract would not absorb the drug even if it's in the milk. (Pharmacology; General Principles; Knowledge; Difficulty 5)

10.   The answer is A. Colostrum is the treatment of choice for asymptomatic hypoglycemia. A small amount of colostrum stabilizes blood sugar. Some methods of testing blood sugar are not accurate. Direct breastfeeding is always the first and best course of action. A newborn normally breastfeeds every 1 to 3 hours in the first 24 hours, and nothing in this question indicates when, if ever, the baby had previously been fed. (Pathology; 1 to 2 days; Application; Difficulty 4)

11.   The answer is D. No assumptions can be made about her ability to breastfeed after breast surgery, although she should be followed closely in the first week postbirth because surgery can disrupt ducts and nerve pathways needed for adequate milk synthesis. (Pathology; Prenatal; Application; Difficulty 3)

12.   The answer is D. Bright red lochia at 14 days with signs of low milk supply suggest that retained placental fragments are suppressing the onset of Lactogenesis II. (Pathology; 3 to 14 days; Application; Difficulty 3)

13.   The answer is B. Allergic disease is responsible for one third of pediatric office visits in the United States. The other statements are true. (Pathology; General Principles; Knowledge; Difficulty 2)

14.   The answer is D. Whether or not she is breastfeeding, a new mother with MS is likely to experience an increase in acute episodes during the postpartum period. Often, breastfeeding is wrongly blamed for this phenomenon. (Pathology; 1 to 2 days; Knowledge; Difficulty 4)

15.   The answer is D. Lumps that do not change size related to milk flow are considered ominous. The mother should be evaluated by a physician immediately. The other characteristics are fairly common during lactation. (Pathology; 15 to 28 days; Application; Difficulty 2)

16.   The answer is B. Mother-baby cross infection is likely when the baby has an oral infection. Assume that the mother's nipples are also infected with the same organism, as well as other infant body parts and any/all sucking objects. (Pathology; 15 to 28 days; Application; Difficulty 3)

17.   The answer is C. Short sucking bursts with pauses are an indicator of immaturity. The other patterns are indicators of a mature infant. (Physiology; Labor/birth (perinatal); Application; Difficulty 2)

18.   The answer is B. Use of progestin-containing contraceptives can diminish milk supply, especially if given prior to 8 weeks postbirth. The other methods do not use hormones and are highly compatible with breastfeeding. (Physiology; 1 to 3 months; Knowledge; Difficulty 2)

19.   The answer is B. There is no evidence that continuing to breastfeed both children is harmful to either child or the mother. (Physiology; 3 to 14 days; Application; Difficulty 3)

20. The answer is D. Stools of young, exclusively breastfed babies are exactly as described and pictured. (Physiology; 15 to 28 days; Application; Difficulty 3)

21. The answer is B. The release of cholecystokinin causes satiety and relaxation. (Physiology; General Principles; Knowledge; Difficulty 2)

22. The answer is D. Libido varies widely among breastfeeding women. Men/fathers should be helped to find new ways to please the mother that are compatible to the biology and psychology of the breastfeeding period. (Physiology; 1 to 3 months; Application; Difficulty 3)

23. The answer is D. When baby is exclusively breastfeeding day and night without long periods away from the breast, the baby is under 6 months old, and the mother's menses have not returned, there is only a 1% to 2% chance of pregnancy at this time. (Physiology; 4 to 6 months; Knowledge; Difficulty 3)

24. The answer is D. Lactogenesis II, or the onset of copius milk secretion, is not dependent on breast stimulation by the baby. All the other statements are true. (Physiology; Labor/birth (perinatal); Knowledge; Difficulty 3)

25. The answer is D. Long periods without collecting milk will cause milk stasis, which will suppress lactogenesis II. Frequent and thorough removal of milk is essential. (Physiology; Prematurity; Application; Difficulty 5)

26. The answer is D. The most important regulatory mechanism for milk synthesis is frequent and thorough milk removal. (Physiology; 15 to 28 days; Application; Difficulty 4)

27. The answer is A. Gut closure occurs around 6 months in the full-term baby. The risk of allergic sensitization from bovine protein is higher before gut closure. (Physiology; 7 to 12 months; Application; Difficulty 4)

28. The answer is C. The nipple tip extends to or close to the juncture of the hard and soft palates during normal latch and positioning. (Anatomy; 1 to 2 days; Application; Difficulty 4)

29. The answer is B. Smooth muscle fibers are found in the nipple-areola complex. (Anatomy; General Principles; Knowledge; Difficulty 3)

30. The answer is A. Left occiput anterior (LOA) is the most common fetal presentation and least likely to cause birth trauma which could affect a baby's ability to breastfeed. Posterior presentations are less common; mentum and sacrum presentations are rare. (Anatomy; Prenatal; Application; Difficulty 2)

31. The answer is D. The other areas may have extra mammary and/or nipple tissue, which are remnants of the galactic band. (Anatomy; Preconception; Knowledge; Difficulty 3)

32.   The answer is C. Undetected breast cancer is very unlikely this early postbirth. Any birth injury may be painful for the baby. Placing the sore side higher than the normal side may reduce pain, resulting in the baby's strong preference for the more comfortable position. Breasts differ in configuration, and one may be easier for the baby to manage in the early weeks. (Anatomy; 15 to 28 days; Application; Difficulty 2)

33.   The answer is A. The infant's epiglottis covers the trachea during swallowing, preventing milk from entering the airway. Between swallows, it prevents air from entering the esophagus. (Anatomy; General Principles; Knowledge; Difficulty 4)

34.   The answer is C. Growth of the secretory epithelial cells is the primary factor causing breast growth during pregnancy. (Anatomy; Prenatal; Application; Difficulty 5)

35.   The answer is B. Cooper's ligaments support the breasts. Softening or stretching of these ligaments during pregnancy many contribute to sagging (Anatomy; Prenatal; Knowledge; Difficulty 3)

36.   The answer is D. The mesenteric nodes are in the abdomen. The other nodes are major collecting points for lymph from the breast area. (Anatomy; General Principles; Knowledge; Difficulty 5)

37.   The answer is B. Macrophages and possibly neutrophils and T-lymphocytes actively kill microbes by phagocytosis. (Biochemistry; General Principles; Knowledge; Difficulty 5)

38.   The answer is D. Breastfeeding triggers and enhances maturation of the baby's own immune system. (Immunology; General Principles; Application; Difficulty 5)

39.   The answer is C. Menstrual irregularities and pain are not known to be related to whether the woman breastfed her children. (Immunology; Preconception; Knowledge; Difficulty 2)

40.   The answer is C. Protection against many short- and long-term diseases is well established, even though the specific mechanisms are still poorly understood as of this writing. (Immunology; >12 months; Knowledge; Difficulty 3)

41.   The answer is B. As of this writing, a link between osteoarthritis and artificial feeding has not been demonstrated in the literature. Eczema is strongly related to artificial feeding; ulcerative colitis and respiratory infections are associated with artificial feeding. (Immunology; >12 months; Knowledge; Difficulty 4)

42.   The answer is A. The mother's milk contains rubella-specific antibodies within 48 hours of maternal exposure. The baby has already been exposed, therefore continued breastfeeding helps protect the baby. (Immunology; 1 to 3 months; Application; Difficulty 3)

43.   The answer is C. The biochemical, physical, immunological, and neurodevelopmental effects of breastfeeding and lactation forever change the mother and baby. (Immunology; General Principles; Knowledge; Difficulty 3)

44. The answer is A. As of this writing, no relationship between breast-feeding and the risk of cervical cancer has been investigated. The risk for all of the others are higher for women who do not breastfeed/lactate. (Immunology; General Principles; Knowledge; Difficulty 4)

45. The answer is B. Breastmilk optimizes the environment in the baby's gut. Allergens may be present in breastmilk and may create problems for a sensitive baby, but the risk of allergies is significantly reduced through breastfeeding. (Immunology; 15 to 28 days; Application; Difficulty 4)

46. The answer is B. Keeping the dyad together is the most supportive action. (Pathology; 15 to 28 days; Application; Difficulty 4)

47. The answer is C. The foramen ovale may remain open or be re-opened by excessive infant crying, which produces a Valsalva effect and increases thoracic pressure. (Anatomy; Prenatal; Application; Difficulty 5)

48. The answer is B. Lactoferrin has no known function relative to nerve growth. It is a major protein source, iron transport agent, and reduces/prevents inflammation. (Biochemistry; General Principles; Knowledge; Difficulty 5)

49. The answer is A. Epidermal growth factor plays a major role in gut maturation. Lactoferrin also promotes tissue maturation. (Biochemistry; General Principles; Knowledge; Difficulty 5)

50. The answer is B. SigA may be targeted to a specific pathogen, but does not directly kill bacteria. (Biochemistry; General Principles; Knowledge; Difficulty 2)

51. The answer is C. Manufacturers are experimenting with the addition of nucleotides to increase the protective properties of their products. However, even with nucleotides added, the manufactured products fall far short of human milk's protective properties. (Biochemistry; General Principles; Knowledge; Difficulty 2)

52. The answer is B. Human milk is 99% bioavailable to the infant, leaving very little residue in the gut. (Biochemistry; General Principles; Knowledge; Difficulty 2)

53. The answer is B. Amniotic fluid provides protein and other nutrients to the fetus in addition to nutrients present in the cord blood vessels. (Biochemistry; Prenatal; Knowledge; Difficulty 3)

54. The answer is A. Immune factors form a layer in milk that is the first to appear in the colostral phase and the last to disappear during weaning. Some factors even increase over time. (Biochemistry; General Principles; Knowledge; Difficulty 3)

55. The answer is B. Only about 500 calories from her diet are used in making milk. (Biochemistry; Prenatal; Knowledge; Difficulty 2)

56. The answer is A. She needs a dietary source of calcium, which is high in all of the choices except rice and potatoes. (Biochemistry; General Principles; Knowledge; Difficulty 2)

57. The answer is B. The Code specifies that information on artificial feeding provided to health workers should be scientific and accurate. Detailed accurate information on product composition, provided to health workers, is appropriate marketing of products within the scope of the Code. (Public Health; General Principles; Knowledge; Difficulty 2)

58. The answer is A. Preterm milk is similar to term milk in lactose, phosphorus, iron and most other components. (Biochemistry; Prematurity; Knowledge; Difficulty 4)

59. The answer is A. Lactose does not appear to be protective against inflammation or pathogens. Fatty acids disrupt cell membranes of some viruses. Lysozyme kills bacteria by disrupting cell walls. Mucins adhere to pathogens, preventing their attachment to mucous membranes. (Biochemistry; General Principles; Application; Difficulty 5)

60. The answer is D. The visual system is the last sensory system to develop during gestation, therefore the most affected by preterm nutrition. Human milk makes a significant difference in visual development of the preterm infant, partly because of fatty acid profiles. (Biochemistry; Prematurity; Knowledge; Difficulty 2)

61. The answer is C. Docosahexanoic acid is a long-chain fatty acid which is found in the fatty portion of milk, not the whey portion. (Biochemistry; General Principles; Knowledge; Difficulty 2)

62. The answer is B. A vegan diet includes no animal sources and is thus deficient in Vitamin B12. A supplement taken by the mother will provide adequate B12 to the baby through her milk. (Biochemistry; Prenatal; Application; Difficulty 4)

63. The answer is B. As of this writing, donor milk has not been prescribed for skin treatment of burns. (Equipment; General Principles; Knowledge; Difficulty 5)

64. The answer is C. Research has established that a premature baby can go to breast safely earlier than he can feed from devices. (Equipment; Prematurity; Application; Difficulty 2)

65. The answer is A. Increased carrying when the baby is not fussy as well as when he is fussy reduces total crying per day. (Equipment; Prematurity; Knowledge; Difficulty 2)

66. The answer is D. Bottle-feeding has been shown to be stressful for preterm infants and increases the risks of premature weaning. (Equipment; Prematurity; Application; Difficulty 5)

67. The answer is C. Her breast reduction surgery may have severed the nerves and ducts needed for adequate lactation. Close follow-up is essential. (Equipment; 1 to 2 days; Application; Difficulty 3)

68. The answer is C. The lactation consultant supports the breastfeeding relationship, including helping the mother to explore all her options in any given situation. (Techniques; 1 to 3 months; Application; Difficulty 2)

69. The answer is C. Assessing the dyad's current feeding patterns is the first step. After that, the other strategies may be appropriate. (Techniques; 3 to 14 days; Knowledge; Difficulty 4)

70. The answer is B. Artificial feeding carries substantial risks that are only exaggerated by the infant's vulnerability to upper respiratory infection. (Techniques; 3 to 14 days; Application; Difficulty 2)

71. The answer is B. Living cells, including macrophages, are killed by freezing. The other components are not significantly affected by freezing. (Techniques; General Principles; Knowledge; Difficulty 2)

72. The answer is C. Fats are most difficult for preterms to digest. Human milk fat is released simultaneously with digestive enzymes, making it optimal for preterms. (Physiology; Prematurity; Knowledge; Difficulty 4)

73. The answer is C. Both groups had the same care (or lack of care) before the study period began. The other choices are all significant flaws. (Research; 15 to 28 days; Application; Difficulty 5)

74. The answer is B. Comparing breastfeeding with artificial feeding suggests their equivalence, which is neither accurate nor helpful information. (Research; General Principles; Knowledge; Difficulty 2)

75. The answer is B. The median score is the middle score, which may or may not also be the mean (average) or mode (most frequent) score. (Research; General Principles; Knowledge; Difficulty 3)

76. The answer is A. The probability of a chance occurrence is 1.0. The smaller the probability value, the LEAST likely the event happened by chance. (Research; General Principles; Knowledge; Difficulty 3)

77. The answer is D. A research article published in a peer-reviewed professional journal is a primary reference. A is a review article, which is a secondary reference. B is a chapter in a book, which is a secondary or tertiary source. C is a book for parents, interpreting other sources in its recommendations. (Research; Prematurity; Application; Difficulty 4)

78. The answer is B. Clinical services are considered breastfeeding support, not promotion. The other activities are considered advocacy or promotion. (Public Health; General Principles; Knowledge; Difficulty 2)

79. The answer is D. Education provided by sources with a conflict of interest is inappropriate and is likely to be inaccurate and unhelpful. (Public Health; General Principles; Knowledge; Difficulty 2)

80. The answer is D. Involving all pertinent staff, planning sufficient education, and providing substantial evidence of the safety and effectiveness of the new policy are all successful strategies for changing policies. Forcing new policies on staff is likely to result in open and covert resistance. (Public Health; 1 to 2 days; Application; Difficulty 2)

81.   The answer is C. The ILO conventions do not specifically address on-site child care. On-site child care is beneficial to all parents, especially breastfeeding mothers. (Public Health; General Principles; Knowledge; Difficulty 2)

82.   The answer is C. The Baby Friendly Hospital Initiative, Step 9, is "Give no artificial teats or pacifiers (also called dummies or soothers) to breastfeeding infants." This Step also includes prohibition of feeding bottles. (Public Health; 1 to 2 days; Knowledge; Difficulty 2)

83.   The answer is D. Direct breastfeeding is the norm. All other feeding methods are considered interventions with known and unknown consequences. (Legal; General Principles; Knowledge; Difficulty 3)

84.   The answer is B. Taking a thorough history is top priority when solving a breastfeeding problem. It is highly likely that the baby is having an allergic reaction to the large amount of milk consumed by the mother. (Techniques; General Principles; Application; Difficulty 3)

85.   The answer is A. Consent must be obtained before touching the mother or baby, or taking photographs. Unwanted touching could be considered battery. Written consent is preferred over verbal. (Legal; General Principles; Knowledge; Difficulty 2)

86.   The answer is C. Referring to one's self is a conflict of interest. (Legal; 3 to 14 days; Knowledge; Difficulty 4)

87.   The answer is B. Malpractice insurance companies have a team of attorneys to represent their clients in legal matters. (Legal; General Principles; Application; Difficulty 4)

88.   The answer is D. Active listening is the FIRST action because the mother is obviously emotionally upset. Understanding, addressing, and exploring feelings is key to counseling the breastfeeding mother. (Psychology; 1 to 3 months; Application; Difficulty 4)

89.   The answer is A. Mothers of multiples most often attach to the unit before the individual baby/babies. (Psychology; General Principles; Knowledge; Difficulty 4)

90.   The answer is B. Employee productivity is actually increased when mothers are enabled to continue breastfeeding their babies. (Psychology; General Principles; Knowledge; Difficulty 2)

91.   The answer is A. Closely supervised breastfeeding may help her. The key is close supervision to protect her and her baby. (Psychology; General Principles; Knowledge; Difficulty 2)

92.   The answer is B. Application of noxious substances to the nipples to discourage breastfeeding can disrupt the trust relationship that has been carefully established via breastfeeding. The other suggestions are appropriate. (Psychology; >12 months; Application; Difficulty 2)

93.   The answer is B. Mothers who breastfeed often want to tell the world, which is a strong theme of empowerment. (Psychology; General Principles; Knowledge; Difficulty 3)

94. The answer is C. Research shows that mothers are reliable witnesses and reporters of their babies' conditions, and sudden disinterest in breastfeeding may indicate a significant problem in the baby. (Psychology; General Principles; Application; Difficulty 3)

95. The answer is B. Beginning your interaction with an empathetic response such as B helps validate the mother's emotions, helps her integrate her experience, and moves her into problem solving. (Psychology; 3 to 14 days; Application; Difficulty 4)

96. The answer is D. Rooming-in enhances the mother-baby relationship and has no known detrimental effect on relationships with grandparents. (Psychology; Labor/birth (perinatal); Knowledge; Difficulty 2)

97. The answer is A. The first statement to the mother should be a positive statement. Afterward, a fuller explanation of induced lactation should take place, which might include any or all of the other choices. (Psychology; 1 to 3 months; Application; Difficulty 2)

98. The answer is A. Crying is a late sign of hunger after all other cues have been ignored. (Growth; 1 to 2 days; Application; Difficulty 2)

99. The answer is D. Breastfed babies initially gain more weight, then by 12 months are leaner per height than artificially fed babies. (Growth; General Principles; Knowledge; Difficulty 3)

100. The answer is A. This a normal pattern. (Growth; 15 to 28 days; Knowledge; Difficulty 2)

101. The answer is D. Babies have individual needs that are best met by feedings on cue, day and night, until they outgrow the need. (Growth; 4 to 6 months; Application; Difficulty 3)

102. The answer is D. Nursing strikes are indications that the baby is having some difficulty with breastfeeding or there is a problem in the mother-baby breastfeeding relationship. Self-weaning before 12 months of age is unusual. (Growth; 7 to 12 months; Application; Difficulty 2)

103. The answer is C. Persistent milk stasis is the chief cause of suppressed lactation (inadequate milk supply). Frequent, thorough removal of milk is necessary to sustain lactation. The other factors listed are old myths and not central to maintaining milk synthesis. (Physiology; 3 to 14 days; Knowledge; Difficulty 5)

104. The answer is B. Extended breastfeeding for more than 2 years has no documented risks for mother or baby, and many benefits for both. (Growth; >12 months; Knowledge; Difficulty 3)

105. The answer is C. Distractability is a common behavioral characteristic of the 4 to 6 month age. (Growth; 4 to 6 months; Knowledge; Difficulty 3)

106. The answer is D. The Babinski reflex, flaring of the toes, is triggered when the sole of the foot is stimulated. (Physiology; 1 to 2 days; Knowledge; Difficulty 4)

107. The answer is D. Steroids do not reduce the infant's risk of allergy and have other consequences. The other strategies will help postpone the onset and/or delay the severity of allergic disease in her child. (Immunology; Prenatal; Application; Difficulty 2)

108. The answer is A. Effective, exclusive breastfeeding does not result in growth faltering. (Pathology; 4 to 6 months; Application; Difficulty 2)

109. The answer is C. The infant gut takes up to 2 weeks to recover from damage caused by a reaction to a single bottle of artificial baby milk. (Immunology; 1 to 2 days; Knowledge; Difficulty 4)

110. The answer is C. The mother's activity is the least likely to cause a problem with initiation of breastfeeding of the second-born twin. (Pathology; Labor and birth; Application; Difficulty 3)

111. The answer is C. The baby may breastfeed normally. Maternal thyroid disease that is properly treated is compatible with breastfeeding. (Pathology; 1 to 2 days; Knowledge; Difficulty 3)

112. The answer is D. Babies with galactosemia cannot metabolize lactose, which is in high amounts in human milk. If the inability to metabolize lactose is complete, the baby cannot have any breastmilk at all. (Pathology; 1 to 2 days; Knowledge; Difficulty 4)

113. The answer is B. The baby should be allowed to feed in his own preferred pattern, which may be one breast per feed or even several feeds on one breast before switching to the other. Getting too little fat-rich hindmilk is one cause of rapid weight gain with fussy, gassy behavior. (Pathology; 15 to 28 days; Application; Difficulty 4)

114. The answer is C. The Baby Friendly Hospital Initiative is designed to protect breastfed babies from practices and policies that disrupt or interfere with breastfeeding. (Public Health; 1 to 2 days; Knowledge; Difficulty 4)

115. The answer is D. White cells in milk do not directly attack dietary allergens. The other answers are true. (Immunology; General Principles; Knowledge; Difficulty 2)

116. The answer is D. The alveoli are positioned back in the breast tissue, and rarely are inside the baby's mouth. A portion of the areola should be inside the infant's mouth, but not necessarily all of it, depending on the areola diameter. A portion of the lactiferous sinuses will be inside the baby's mouth (Anatomy; 1 to 2 days; Application; Difficulty 2)

117. The answer is C. Holder pasteurization for human milk banks raises milk to 62.5 degrees Celsius for 30 minutes. (Equipment; General Principles; Knowledge; Difficulty 5)

118. The answer is A. Exclusive breastfeeding means that the baby satisfies all nutrition and sucking at his mother's breast. Option B has use of devices; Option C includes other fluids, and Option D could include other fluids and/or pacifiers. (Legal; General Principles; Knowledge; Difficulty 5)

119. The answer is C. About 1% of most medications given to a lactating woman actually gets to her breastfed baby. (Pharmacology; General Principles; Knowledge; Difficulty 3)

120. The answer is C. Antineoplastics are used in treating malignant tumors. Breastfeeding is usually contraindicated because of the potential risk to the infant. (Pharmacology; General Principles; Knowledge; Difficulty 4)

121. The answer is B. Perineally injected medications transfer to the infant poorly if at all. (Pharmacology; Labor/birth (perinatal); Application; Difficulty 5)

122. The answer is B. Milk ducts sometimes terminate on the areola, causing milk to be released during the milk ejection reflex. This is a normal breast configuration. (Anatomy; 3 to 14 days; Knowledge; Difficulty 3)

123. The answer is B. Mother-baby cross-infection is likely when the baby has an oral infection. Assume that the mother's nipples are also infected with the same organism, as well as other infant body parts and any/all sucking objects. (Pathology; 1 to 3 months; Application; Difficulty 2)

124. The answer is C. The peaked shape does not "look good"—it suggests a shallow latch and/or poor sucking technique, both of which need attention and correction. A, B, and D are all reasonable and appropriate suggestions. (Pathology; 15 to 28 days; Application; Difficulty 2)

125. The answer is B. The baby is being treated for hyperbilirubinemia. If this appears in the first 24 to 48 hours, the most likely cause is ABO incompatibility. (Pathology; 1 to 2 days; Knowledge; Difficulty 2)

126. The answer is C. This flat nipple has damage on the face (front) surface extending onto the top edge, visible as a darker red color on the extreme right vertical edge. The baby was tongue-tied, exacerbating the abrasion of the nipple tip on the palate. Other nipple characteristics can't be assessed visually. (Pathology; 15 to 28 days; Application; Difficulty 3)

127. The answer is A. Observing a breastfeed is the first step in identifying the cause of painful nipples. (Pathology; 3 to 14 days; Application; Difficulty 3)

128. The answer is C. Expressing or pumping milk may be helpful if a breast abscess is so close to the nipple that the baby cannot effectively feed. The other conditions are compatible with continued breastfeeding. (Pathology; 1 to 3 months; Knowledge; Difficulty 3)

129. The answer is A. The nipple is normal shape and the breast is not full post-feed. Both of these suggest maternal comfort with effective milk transfer. If milk transfer was poor, there should be breast fullness post-feed. If the mother experienced pain, there is usually nipple distortion visible post-feed. (Techniques; 3 to 14 days; Application; Difficulty 3)

130. The answer is D. Determination of sufficient or insufficient glandular tissue for lactation cannot be determined by physical examination alone. This woman breastfed each of her two children for over 2 years each. (Techniques; General Principles; Application; Difficulty 5)

131. The answer is A. This is milk residue. The mother had just finished pumping her milk. (Pathology; 3 to 14 days; Application; Difficulty 4)

132. The answer is B. This is a large, fibrous nipple with no abnormal conditions. (Pathology; 3 to 14 days; Knowledge; Difficulty 4)

133. The answer is C. The dark marks are bruises from her baby's off-center latch. The photo was taken on day 3. (Pathology; 3 to 14 days; Application; Difficulty 4)

134. The answer is D. Reinforcing the mother is the first strategy to support her decision and build confidence. After rapport is established, attending to the baby's possible jaundice and breastfeeding management questions is appropriate. (Pathology; 3 to 14 days; Application; Difficulty 4)

135. The answer is B. Supine sleeping is strongly associated with lower risk of sudden infant death syndrome. This position also makes breastfeeding at night easier. (Pathology; 1 to 3 months; Knowledge; Difficulty 2)

136. The answer is B. The baby's skin is slightly yellow, suggesting hyperbilirubinemia. Assuring frequent, effective breastfeeds is the most appropriate strategy to use at this point. (Pathology; 1 to 2 days; Application; Difficulty 4)

137. The answer is B. As this child naturally explores his environment, he is exposed to many more pathogens. Some immune components of human milk increase over time. (Pathology; 4 to 6 months; Application; Difficulty 4)

138. The answer is D. Biting during nursing is not likely to cause a wound in this position—it is more likely to cause a wound at the nipple-areola juncture. The other causes are quite possible. In this mother's case, the baby had a shallow latch, which was quickly and easily corrected. (Pathology; 3 to 14 days; Application; Difficulty 5)

139. The answer is C. Providing medications is not within the current scope of practice of the Lactation Consultant. The other actions are appropriate. (Pathology; 4 to 6 months; Application; Difficulty 4)

140.   The answer is D. The location of the abrasions suggest that the baby is nursing on the nipple tips instead of taking a large, deep grasp of the nipple/areola complex. (Physiology; 15 to 28 days; Application; Difficulty 5)

141.   The answer is B. Babies should be breastfed when they show signs of hunger. Crying, as shown in the picture, is a LATE hunger cue. The other options do not meet the baby's need for frequent feedings. (Physiology; 15 to 28 days; Application; Difficulty 3)

142.   The answer is B. The BFHI recommends that the baby breastfeed within 30 to 60 minutes after birth. (Physiology; Labor/birth (perinatal); Knowledge; Difficulty 3)

143.   The answer is D. The compression stripe from 1:00 to 7:00 indicates a shallow latch. The first intervention should be correcting the positioning and latch during feeds. (Physiology; 3 to 14 days; Application; Difficulty 5)

144.   The answer is C. This baby is nearing the end of the feed on this breast and should be allowed to self-detach at his own pace. He is correctly positioned. (Physiology; 15 to 28 days; Application; Difficulty 4)

145.   The answer is D. The swelling is accessory breast tissue that is producing milk in the immediate postbirth period. (Physiology; 3 to 14 days; Knowledge; Difficulty 5)

146.   The answer is A. Kangaroo care, or skin-to-skin contact preserves infant energy as well as the other results listed. It is especially beneficial for premature infants. (Physiology; 1 to 2 days; Knowledge; Difficulty 3)

147.   The answer is B. Many mothers experience tender nipples if they become pregnant while breastfeeding, which appears to be caused by pregnancy hormones. (Physiology; Prenatal; Application; Difficulty 3)

148.   The answer is B. Normal 4-month old babies take an average of 80% of the available milk over the course of the day. Adding complementary foods is no longer recommended; neither are routine vitamin D supplements. The highest risk of SIDS is at 2 to 4 months. (Physiology; 4 to 6 months; Knowledge; Difficulty 4)

149.   The answer is C. The string-like structure connecting the tongue to the floor of the mouth is the lingual frenulum (or frenum). The labial frenulum is on the upper (maxillary) gum ridge. The incisive papilla are behind the upper gum ridge, and mucus membrane covers most of the inside of the baby's mouth. (Anatomy; General Principles; Knowledge; Difficulty 4)

150.   The answer is B. The white objects in this newborn's mouth are natal teeth. (Anatomy; 1 to 2 days; Knowledge; Difficulty 3)

151.   The answer is D. This baby's oral anatomy is normal. (Anatomy; 3 to 14 days; Knowledge; Difficulty 3)

152. The answer is C. The lumps are Montgomery's tubercles (Montgomery glands) and are entirely normal. (Anatomy; 7 to 12 months; Knowledge; Difficulty 3)

153. The answer is C. Nipple preparation has not been shown to be helpful. This wound was caused by a baby whose lingual frenulum was short and tight (tongue-tied). (Anatomy; Prenatal; Application; Difficulty 3)

154. The answer is C. This baby's labial (upper) frenulum is normal. However, the other three choices are possible factors in the baby's clicking and smacking during breastfeeding. The buccal pads are exceptionally prominent. (Anatomy; 1 to 3 months; Application; Difficulty 5)

155. The answer is C. This is mechanical (friction) damage from a tongue-tied baby. A and B do not cause open wounds. D is an old myth, not consistent with current knowledge and research evidence. (Pathology; 1 to 2 days; Application; Difficulty 2)

156. The answer is D. This is an accessory nipple on the woman's upper, inner thigh. This woman found the sensitivity of the skin paralleled her menstrual cycles. (Anatomy; Preconception; Knowledge; Difficulty 4)

157. The answer is C. This woman's large breasts are normal; she has accessory mammary tissue in both axilla. This photo was taken on day 4 postbirth. (Anatomy; 3 to 14 days; Knowledge; Difficulty 5)

158. The answer is B. The baby's short, tight frenulum is restricting proper tongue movement needed for latch and feeding. (Anatomy; 3 to 14 days; Application; Difficulty 4)

159. The answer is A. The baby is entirely healthy and thriving except for an allergic diaper rash caused by dairy in her mother's diet. The other options are inappropriate and incorrect. (Immunology; 15 to 28 days; Application; Difficulty 2)

160. The answer is B. The crack at the base of the nipple was caused by a bacterial infection of her nipple and occurred simultaneously with her baby having a streptococcal infection of the throat. (Immunology; 4 to 6 months; Application; Difficulty 5)

161. The answer is C. Mothers milk contains traces of flavors present in the mother's food choices, which helps the baby learn and enjoy family food preferences. Shortly after this picture was taken, the baby's breath smelled faintly of cantaloupe. (Biochemistry; 3 to 14 days; Application; Difficulty 3)

162. The answer is A. Nursing supplementers were designed to provide food at breast for an adopted baby so that the baby's sucking will help stimulate the mother's breast to make milk. (Equipment; 1 to 3 months; Application; Difficulty 4)

163. The answer is A. Breastfed babies are often willing to try a different feeding method when they are not ravenously hungry. (Equipment; 7 to 12 months; Application; Difficulty 3)

164. The answer is C. The mother can breastfeed directly if she has nipple thrush. All of the other answers are appropriate uses for cup-feeding. (Equipment; 3 to 14 days; Application; Difficulty 2)

165. The answer is D. Mothers with large breasts may enjoy the support of a well-fitting bra. There is no pathology shown in this picture—the baby is nursing well on day 4 postbirth. (Equipment; 3 to 14 days; Application; Difficulty 4)

166. The answer is A. The pumping pattern should closely mimic the baby's feeding pattern of about 40 to 60 cycles of alternating vacuum and release per minute. (Equipment; 3 to 14 days; Application; Difficulty 3)

167. The answer is B. An oral exam is considered a basic lactation assessment. Suck training is considered an advanced therapy and is rarely needed. During fingerfeeding, a thin tube is held against the adult's finger. The baby in the picture is being held and appears asleep; therefore D is unlikely. (Techniques; 1 to 2 days; Application; Difficulty 5)

168. The answer is B. The baby's head is too extended relative to his trunk, so pulling the legs closer to mother will align hip and shoulders. Supporting the breast will not correct the infant's position. The horizontal position and use of a pillow are not likely to help. (Techniques; 15 to 28 days; Application; Difficulty 2)

169. The answer is A. Attempting a deeper latch is the first and usually most effective intervention. If that does not eliminate the pain and result in better feeding, further investigation is needed. (Techniques; 3 to 14 days; Application; Difficulty 4)

170. The answer is A. Deep puckering suggests poor tongue position or motion. In this case, the baby was tongue-tied. Feeding with the eyes closed is a lesser indicator of a problem. The chin and nose are well-positioned. (Techniques; 3 to 14 days; Application; Difficulty 3)

171. The answer is C. Birth injuries such as this wound from a vacuum extractor may cause head pain in the baby. Direct breastfeeding should be tried first; if unsuccessful, other methods could be explored. (Techniques; 1 to 2 days; Application; Difficulty 2)

172. The answer is B. The most likely explanation for sudden onset soreness is poor positioning, causing pulling or tugging on the nipple skin. The first intervention would be correcting positioning and latch. The other choices are possibilities after poor positioning has been ruled out. (Techniques; 4 to 6 months; Application; Difficulty 5)

173. The answer is D. There is no indication for interrupting breastfeeding in this situation. The rash could be bacterial, yeast, eczema, or some other organic condition. A, B, and C are all appropriate suggestions. (Techniques; 4 to 6 months; Application; Difficulty 3)

174.   The answer is C. Radiant warmers do not facilitate maternal access to the infant. Separation from the mother creates psychological and physical stress to the infant, including increased crying, more risk of hypothermia, and release of stress hormones. (Techniques; Labor/birth (perinatal); Application; Difficulty 4)

175.   The answer is B. The most effective treatment for a plugged nipple pore, also known as a "bleb" or "white spot," is softening the plugged area in warm water, then massaging or expressing the duct opening. Hand-expressing before feeds is a technique for softening the entire breast; wearing shells does not treat a plugged pore, and there is no other indication of nipple thrush in this mother's situation. (Techniques; 4 to 6 months; Application; Difficulty 4)

176.   The answer is C. Supporting this soft breast from underneath is the MOST helpful suggestion. This mother's areolae are very large and may not be fully covered by the baby's mouth. Removing the bra is not necessary. Leaning forward is usually uncomfortable at best. (Techniques; 1 to 2 days; Application; Difficulty 3)

177.   The answer is A. Teaching her how to position her baby for breast-feeding is the most important action. Her nipples are not retracted, so B and C are incorrect. Rubbing the skin with rough fabric is inappropriate and can damage areolar structures. (Techniques; Prenatal; Application; Difficulty 4)

178.   The answer is D. The hand positions shown are adequate. The next appropriate action is bringing the baby to the breast. (Techniques; 1 to 2 days; Application; Difficulty 5)

179.   The answer is C. The FIRST suggestion to prevent nipple damage is to support the large, pendulous breasts and help the baby attach deeply onto the breast. A nipple shield is not appropriate for this mother. (Techniques; 3 to 14 days; Application; Difficulty 2)

180.   The answer is C. This baby is $4\frac{1}{2}$ months old and is most likely going through a growth spurt. He is too young to need solid foods. Teething and illness are less common reasons for a sudden change in nursing patterns. (Techniques; 4 to 6 months; Application; Difficulty 4)

181.   The answer is D. This mother is hand-expressing her milk, not doing a pinch test on herself. Expressing is more common, although the hand positions are similar. The retracting nipple is not a problem. (Techniques; 3 to 14 days; Knowledge; Difficulty 4)

182.   The answer is C. This 7-day-old baby is relaxed and feeding well from the cup, which is being used correctly. (Techniques; 3 to 14 days; Application; Difficulty 2)

183.   The answer is C. Allowing the baby to set the pace of feeds is most appropriate. This mother has very large breasts, and the baby may even want to feed more than one time from one breast before switching sides. (Techniques; 3 to 14 days; Application; Difficulty 4)

184. The answer is B. Suggestions to correct or improve breastfeeding technique are generally not the FIRST consideration when working with a healthy 6-month-old. Older babies can place themselves in creative postures and still breastfeed effectively. The other questions assume the normalcy of breastfeeding and provide emotional support while obtaining useful data. (Techniques; 4 to 6 months; Application; Difficulty 4)

185. The answer is D. 24-hour rooming-in from birth onward is Step 7 of the Ten Steps to Successful Breastfeeding. (Public Health; Labor/birth (perinatal); Application; Difficulty 2)

186. The answer is B. Sucking need does not substantially change at 7 to 9 months. Using a pacifier may trigger a nursing strike or premature weaning. (Growth; 7 to 12 months; Application; Difficulty 5)

187. The answer is D. Breastfeeding frequently on cue and continuous/frequent carrying fosters all aspects of infant mental and physical development. (Psychology; >12 months; Application; Difficulty 2)

188. The answer is C. Many mothers have more milk than their baby needs in the first 2 weeks. Supply gradually adjusts to baby's needs over the first 6 weeks or so. (Psychology; 3 to 14 days; Application; Difficulty 4)

189. The answer is C. This mother and baby are content, safe, and warm. Keeping the mother and baby in skin-to-skin contact is ideal for stabilizing the baby's systems. Preserving the mother-baby relationship is a primary responsibility of the lactation consultant. Continue observing the dyad; the baby will likely wake to feed soon. (Psychology; Labor/birth (perinatal); Application; Difficulty 2)

190. The answer is D. Identifying with the mothers' feelings rather than offering solutions allows her to think about her options. (Psychology; 15 to 28 days; Application; Difficulty 2)

191. The answer is A. Doula care (the continuous presence of a trained attendant through the entire labor) enhances the husband's (partner's) involvement in birth. Doula care also extends the duration of breastfeeding, shortens labor, reduces cesarean births, and results in less infant asphyxia. (Psychology; Labor/birth (perinatal); Knowledge; Difficulty 2)

192. The answer is A. The developmental milestones characteristic of the 7 to 12 month age include separation anxiety, sleep changes, especially increased night waking, and decreased (not increased) likelihood of self-weaning. (Growth; 7 to 12 months; Application; Difficulty 4)

193. The answer is B. Sleeping through the night is least likely in this age child. "Gymnastic" nursing, pincer grasp and self-feeding, and separation anxiety are typical of the 7 to 12 month old child. (Growth; 7 to 12 months; Application; Difficulty 5)

194. The answer is C. Babies cue, or signal, for their needs to be met. Crying is a LATE sign of hunger; and also a sign that the baby has exhausted all other resources in getting his needs met. (Growth; 3 to 14 days; Application; Difficulty 2)

195. The answer is D. Feeding at night is normal and widely practiced. It is always appropriate to breastfeed in response to the baby's cues, 24 hours a day. (Growth; 4 to 6 months; Application; Difficulty 3)

196. The answer is A. Object permanence emerges in the 4 to 8 month old period. The child can remember her intention even when the object is moved out of visual range. (Growth; 7 to 12 months; Application; Difficulty 3)

197. The answer is A. An infant can imitate the adult's facial expressions shortly after birth. This baby is 4 days old and clearly is imitating the woman's expression. (Growth; 1 to 2 days; Knowledge; Difficulty 4)

198. The answer is B. In the early weeks, babies often feed with closed fists which open and relax as the baby becomes satiated at breast. (Growth; 3 to 14 days; Application; Difficulty 4)

199. The answer is C. These are typical and normal behaviors of breastfeeding children in the 7 to 12 month period. (Growth; 7 to 12 months; Application; Difficulty 3)

200. The answer is D. Continuous/frequent carrying with unrestricted breastfeeding fosters all aspects of infant mental and physical development. (Growth; 1 to 3 months; Knowledge; Difficulty 2)

EXAM B

1. The answer is A. There are several antidepressant medications considered compatible with breastfeeding by the American Academy of Pediatrics. Continuing to breastfeed may help her recover from her illness. (Pharmacology; 3 to 14 days; Application; Difficulty 4)

2. The answer is A. High lipid solubility would increase drug transfer into milk. The other factors would inhibit passage into milk. (Pharmacology; General Principles; Application; Difficulty 2)

3. The answer is D. One half-life is the time it takes for half of the drug to be metabolized. In the first half-life, 20 mg would be metabolized, leaving 20 mg. After the second half-life, half of the remaining 20 mg would be metabolized, leaving 10 mg. After the third half-life, 5 mg would be left. After 4 half-lives, 2.5 mg of the drug would remain. (Pharmacology; General Principles; Application; Difficulty 4)

4. The answer is C. Drugs that are highly absorbable via oral ingestion more easily transfer to breastmilk. The other properties reduce the amount that may get to the baby. (Pharmacology; General Principles; Knowledge; Difficulty 2)

5. The answer is C. Antineoplastics are used in treating malignant tumors. Breastfeeding is usually contraindicated because of the potential risk to the infant. (Pharmacology; General Principles; Knowledge; Difficulty 4)

6. The answer is C. The risk of drug passage into milk is highest in the early postpartum period when the junctures between the mammary secretory epithelial cells are open. After the first week or so, the tight junctures between cells inhibit most drugs from passing into milk. (Pharmacology; 1 to 2 days; Application; Difficulty 4)

7. The answer is D. Alcohol in milk is directly related to levels in maternal serum and does not accumulate in milk. (Pharmacology; General Principles; Knowledge; Difficulty 4)

8. The answer is B. Iodine 131 is a radioactive isotope requiring temporary cessation of breastfeeding. Mother should express her milk to maintain supply until the isotope is out of her system. (Pharmacology; General Principles; Knowledge; Difficulty 5)

9. The answer is B. Herbal teas may contain substances that exert a pharmacological effect on the baby. (Pharmacology; 15 to 28 days; Knowledge; Difficulty 4)

10. The answer is C. Unresolved stress from the birth can trigger or exacerbate postpartum depression. She needs to see her primary care provider immediately for thorough evaluation, diagnosis, and treatment. (Pathology; 1 to 3 months; Knowledge; Difficulty 4)

11. The answer is D. The U.S. Centers for Disease Control and Prevention does not require health care workers to wear gloves when assisting breastfeeding except in high-exposure situations such as donor milk banking. (Pathology; General Principles; Knowledge; Difficulty 5)

12. The answer is C. Intraductal papilloma is the most likely cause of painless bright red bleeding in the early postpartum period. (Pathology; 1 to 2 days; Knowledge; Difficulty 4)

13. The answer is C. Mothers with diabetes may need less insulin during lactation. Careful monitoring is essential. (Pathology; Prenatal; Application; Difficulty 2)

14. The answer is C. The only limiting factor to breastfeeding is the mother's injuries. Compatible pain medications are available. She and her baby still need each other while she recovers. (Pathology; 4 to 6 months; Application; Difficulty 4)

15. The answer is A. Preterm milk is similar to term milk in lactose, phosphorus, iron, and most other components. (Biochemistry; Prematurity; Knowledge; Difficulty 2)

16. The answer is B. Research shows that babies separated from their mothers are in a state of higher stress. (Pathology; Labor/birth (perinatal); Knowledge; Difficulty 4)

17. The answer is C. Babies feed for varying lengths and at varying intervals according to their hunger, emotional needs, growth and developmental stages, and other physiological factors. Placing restrictions on length or frequency, or offering "substitutes" disrupts the breastfeeding relationship and interferes with fulfillment of infant needs. (Physiology; 1 to 3 months; Application; Difficulty 2)

18. The answer is B. Premature babies often exhibit an irregular and arrhythmic sucking pattern, which improves as they mature. (Physiology; Prematurity; Application; Difficulty 2)

19. The answer is C. Proper sucking is unrelated to urogenital development, but is involved in development of the other systems listed. (Physiology; General Principles; Application; Difficulty 3)

20. The answer is B. Use of progestin-containing contraceptives can diminish milk supply if given prior to 8 weeks postbirth. (Physiology; 1 to 3 months; Knowledge; Difficulty 4)

21. The answer is C. Prolonged elevated bilirubin in a healthy, thriving baby at the level listed is not considered pathological. Continued appropriate breastfeeding practices are the BEST suggestions. (Physiology; 3 to 14 days; Application; Difficulty 3)

22. The answer is C. Longer nursing sessions is MOST likely, although a baby who was recently hospitalized may also nurse more frequently, but not necessarily to quench thirst. It is highly unlikely that a child would want the same or less frequent breastfeeding than prior to the hospitalization. (Physiology; 4 to 6 months; Application; Difficulty 4)

23. The answer is B. Passing black, tarry stools after day 4 is abnormal. The baby needs a thorough medical evaluation to rule out gastro-intestinal bleeding. By day 7, the baby should be passing 3 to 5 or more profuse, loose yellow stools every day. (Physiology; 1 to 2 days; Application; Difficulty 4)

24. The answer is D. Lactocytes (mammary secretory cells, also called glandular tissue) develop on the basement membrane of the duct structure during pregnancy. Growth continues for several weeks postbirth. (Physiology; Prenatal; Knowledge; Difficulty 5)

25. The answer is D. Severe blood loss can cause pituitary shock (Sheehan's syndrome), which blocks prolactin responses needed for lactogenesis III. (Physiology; 3 to 14 days; Knowledge; Difficulty 5)

26. The answer is D. The most important regulatory mechanism for milk synthesis is frequent and thorough milk removal. (Physiology; 15 to 28 days; Application; Difficulty 4)

27. The answer is B. Macrophages and possibly neutrophils and T-lymphocytes actively kill microbes by phagocytosis. (Physiology; Prematurity; Knowledge; Difficulty 4)

28. The answer is C. The sinuses are slight enlargements in the ducts as they near the nipple-areolar complex. Milk-secreting cells are in the alveolus; the areola is possibly a landmark for the baby, and the Montgomery glands (tubercles) secrete a substance that cleanses the areola. (Anatomy; General Principles; Knowledge; Difficulty 3)

29. The answer is C. The tail of Spence is normal mammary glandular tissue extending into the axilla. (Anatomy; General Principles; Knowledge; Difficulty 3)

30. The answer is B. The nipple's sebaceous glands play a very minor, if any, role in lubrication. The nipple is a passageway for milk, probably a visual cue for the baby, and contains many nerve endings involved in the milk-ejection reflex. (Anatomy; General Principles; Application; Difficulty 2)

31. The answer is A. Breast growth (size change) indicates the growth of glandular secretory tissue. Growth patterns may vary widely and still be within normal ranges. Different size breasts are common; expression of colostrum during pregnancy is not expected; and breast shape is rarely relevant to lactation capacity. (Anatomy; Prenatal; Knowledge; Difficulty 3)

32. The answer is C. Normal newborn heart rate is 120 to 160 beats per minute. (Anatomy; Labor/birth (perinatal); Knowledge; Difficulty 5)

33. The answer is A. The mammary ridge forms at 4 to 5 weeks gestation (Anatomy; Preconception; Knowledge; Difficulty 3)

34. The answer is D. The foramen magnum is the large opening in the cranium (skull) through which the spinal cord passes. (Anatomy; Prenatal; Knowledge; Difficulty 2)

35. The answer is A. Caput succedaneum is the collection of fluid between the skin and cranial bone of the newborn, often associated with the use of vacuum extraction devices. Any head injury or insult may affect the infant's ability to breastfeed. (Anatomy; Labor/birth (perinatal); Knowledge; Difficulty 3)

36. The answer is B. The infant develops an immature suck-swallow reflex around 26 weeks gestational age. (Anatomy; Prematurity; Knowledge; Difficulty 4)

37. The answer is D. The lymphatic system drains from the breast tissue; it does not supply components of milk manufacture. (Anatomy; General Principles; Knowledge; Difficulty 2)

38. The answer is A. Short gut syndrome does not appear to be related to infant feeding. All of the others are much more common in those who were artificially fed. (Immunology; General Principles; Knowledge; Difficulty 2)

39. The answer is C. Even tuberculosis may be less of a risk in the breastfed infant. The other diseases are strongly associated with artificial feeding. (Immunology; General Principles; Knowledge; Difficulty 5)

40. The answer is A. Viral fragments in milk do not appear to actually transmit disease from mother to infant. (Immunology; General Principles; Knowledge; Difficulty 2)

41. The answer is B. Professional malpractice insurance companies have a team of attorneys to represent their clients in ethical and legal matters. (Legal; General Principles; Knowledge; Difficulty 3)

42. The answer is D. There is no evidence that the mother will become less ill because she is lactating. Antibodies and white cells that she produces quickly get into her milk and protect the baby. A mother who is sick may be further stressed by the additional work of preparing artificial feeds. (Immunology; 4 to 6 months; Application; Difficulty 2)

43. The answer is A. Exclusive breastfeeding for about 6 months is the best strategy to reduce the baby's risk. The mother's avoidance of known allergens during pregnancy may also reduce the baby's risks of allergy. It is more important that the mother exclusively breastfeed for about 6 months than other actions she should be considering at this time. Delaying solid foods does not address the baby's more likely early exposure to cow's milk and soy proteins, which are very common allergens in humans. (Immunology; Prenatal; Knowledge; Difficulty 3)

44. The answer is C. With very rare exceptions, breastfeeding should continue if the mother is ill at the time of birth or if she becomes ill during breastfeeding. (Immunology; General Principles; Application; Difficulty 3)

45. The answer is B. A good maternal diet during pregnancy significantly reduces the incidence of low birthweight infants. Diet may have a relationship to the development of gestational diabetes. Maternal diet does not directly affect A or D. (Biochemistry; Prenatal; Knowledge; Difficulty 3)

46. The answer is D. Current recommendations are for pregnant women of normal prepregnancy weight to gain at least 25 pounds during pregnancy. Underweight women and teenagers should gain even more weight to sustain their growing bodies and the developing fetus. (Biochemistry; Prenatal; Application; Difficulty 3)

47. The answer is B. Freezing destroys living white cells such as T- and B-lymphocytes. The other components are not significantly affected by freezing. (Biochemistry; General Principles; Knowledge; Difficulty 5)

48. The answer is B. Prostaglandins in the milk have antiinflammatory properties that protect all tissues, especially the infant gut. (Biochemistry; General Principles; Knowledge; Difficulty 4)

49. The answer is A. Ritual feeds increase the risk of infections and illnesses and interfere with breastfeeding. (Biochemistry; 1 to 2 days; Knowledge; Difficulty 5)

50. The answer is D. Bifidus factor supports gut colonization with *Lactobacillus bifidus,* a friendly bacteria that protects the gut mucosa from pathogens. Bifidus factor is not found in the milk of other animals. (Biochemistry; 15 to 28 days; Knowledge; Difficulty 3)

51. The answer is C. Fat-soluble vitamin intake depends on fat levels in milk, which varies with several factors. Protein, minerals, and lactose do not vary with infant feeding patterns. (Biochemistry; General Principles; Knowledge; Difficulty 2)

52. The answer is B. Manufacturers omitted chloride in a mistaken effort to impact adult cardiac disease by changing infant intake of salt. (Biochemistry; General Principles; Knowledge; Difficulty 5)

53. The answer is A. Women who eat no animal products need a dietary source of Vitamin B12. The other nutrients listed can be obtained from plant foods. (Biochemistry; Prenatal; Application; Difficulty 5)

54. The answer is C. Sucrose is not found in human milk. The other carbohydrates play an important role in infant growth and immune function. (Biochemistry; General Principles; Knowledge; Difficulty 3)

55. The answer is B. The most important function of colostrum is to protect the baby from pathogens. Colostrum is especially high in secretory IgA and white cells. (Biochemistry; Labor/birth (perinatal); Knowledge; Difficulty 3)

56. The answer is B. Preterm infants are often unable to absorb iron effectively, and may need supplementation. (Biochemistry; Prematurity; Knowledge; Difficulty 4)

57. The answer is B. Lactose aids absorption of calcium and iron. (Biochemistry; General Principles; Knowledge; Difficulty 5)

58. The answer is A. Milk volumes consumed are relatively stable at 750 to 800 ml/day from the first week or so until at least 6 months. The range can vary widely and still be normal. Babies deliberately leave some milk in the breasts. Artificially fed babies may need more milk as they get older because the nutrients are less available for growth. (Biochemistry; 4 to 6 months; Application; Difficulty 5)

59. The answer is C. Lipase present in human milk digests and breaks down the fatty acids, and may change the taste and smell of stored milk. The stored milk is still safe and healthy for the baby. (Biochemistry; 1 to 3 months; Application; Difficulty 3)

60. The answer is A. The whey-casein ratio changes from 90:10 in the newborn period to closer to 60:40 around 6 months (Biochemistry; 1 to 3 months; Knowledge; Difficulty 3)

61. The answer is A. Calcium is found in artificial feeding products. The other components listed are not found in manufactured foods for infants. (Biochemistry; General Principles; Knowledge; Difficulty 2)

62. The answer is C. Holder pasteurization for human milk banks raises milk to 62.5 degrees Celsius for 30 minutes. (Equipment; General Principles; Knowledge; Difficulty 5)

63. The answer is D. Spoons and open cups are easier to clean than other feeding devices. (Equipment; Prematurity; Application; Difficulty 4)

64. The answer is C. Teats have significant drawbacks, yet in some circumstances can help stimulate a baby's suck response and aid in getting a baby to or back to breast. They should be used only rarely and if other methods fail. (Equipment; Prematurity; Application; Difficulty 2)

65. The answer is C. SigA is stable to heat treatment and freezing. (Equipment; General Principles; Knowledge; Difficulty 5)

66. The answer is B. The least expensive device may not be effective, nor is it necessarily the most appropriate device for the situation. (Equipment; General Principles; Application; Difficulty 2)

67. The answer is A. Breast shells have not been found to be safe and effective for "correcting" non-protractile nipples. The other statements are all appropriate. (Equipment; Prenatal; Application; Difficulty 2)

68. The answer is D. The rolling action presses milk out of the lactiferous sinuses toward the nipple. (Techniques; General Principles; Application; Difficulty 3)

69. The answer is D. Direct breastfeeding should be tried first. Devices should only be considered when direct breastfeeding is impossible. (Techniques; 1 to 2 days; Application; Difficulty 3)

70. The answer is D. The 1- to 3-month-old's feeds are usually spaced throughout the day and night. Clustering is more likely in the late afternoon or early evening. B and C are unusual patterns for a thriving, exclusively breastfed 2-month-old. (Techniques; 1 to 3 months; Knowledge; Difficulty 4)

71. The answer is D. Skin-to-skin contact with reduced sensory stimulation is the FIRST and usually successful intervention. Once that is done, A could help. B is harsh and usually unnecessary. Pulling down a baby's chin may cause jaw clenching. (Techniques; Labor/birth (perinatal); Application; Difficulty 4)

72. The answer is B. Pre and post feed weight checks on a sensitive scale is the most accurate and least disruptive of the options listed. Expressing is disruptive. Weighing the mother and counting swallows are less accurate. (Techniques; 4 to 6 months; Application; Difficulty 4)

73. The answer is D. Case reports are the weakest form of evidence for a given policy or practice. Systematic reviews and meta-analyses are the strongest. (Research; General Principles; Knowledge; Difficulty 2)

74. The answer is C. Original research (primary references) is the most important type of source to include in a literature review. Texts and review articles may help you locate primary references on a subject. Lectures also may direct you to primary references. (Research; General Principles; Application; Difficulty 4)

75. The answer is D. Clinical trials are rarely the first type of research done to investigate a phenomenon. Observational studies, qualitative surveys, and case reports establish the basis for possible later clinical trials. (Research; General Principles; Application; Difficulty 2)

76. The answer is B. The Hawthorne effect means that observing a population for a specific behavior change often produces the desired change, independent of the intervention being studied. (Research; Prenatal; Application; Difficulty 2)

77. The answer is B. Both documents recommend exclusive breastfeeding for about 6 months. (Older documents recommend exclusive breastfeeding for 4 to 6 months.) (Public Health; 4 to 6 months; Knowledge; Difficulty 5)

78. The answer is B. Step 10 of the Baby Friendly Hospital Initiative addresses the importance of referring new mothers to peer support groups. The other actions, although appropriate, are less likely to result in her continuing to breastfeed successfully. (Public Health; 3 to 14 days; Application; Difficulty 5)

79. The answer is D. The fourth provision of the Innocenti Declaration protects the breastfeeding rights of working women, not their right to breastfeed in public. (Public Health; General Principles; Knowledge; Difficulty 2)

80. The answer is C. Family violence has not yet been linked to breast-feeding at the policy level. One study suggests that violence in the home is a barrier to women breastfeeding. (Public Health; General Principles; Knowledge; Difficulty 2)

81. The answer is D. Libido is not addressed in safe mother hood initiatives. Libido is not necessarily lower during breastfeeding. (Public Health; General Principles; Knowledge; Difficulty 2)

82. The answer is A. Breastpumps are not currently covered by the International Code. However, feeding bottles (baby bottles) used as collection containers attached to breast pumps are included in the scope of the code. (Public Health; General Principles; Knowledge; Difficulty 2)

83. The answer is D. All other situations require written documentation. It is preferable to document ALL client and provider contacts. (Legal; General Principles; Knowledge; Difficulty 2)

84. The answer is C. The lactation consultant does not need permission from a physician before assisting a baby with cleft palate to breast-feed. (Legal; General Principles; Knowledge; Difficulty 2)

85. The answer is D. Lactation consultants do not determine the safety of prescribed medications, although they may provide information on compatibility of medications to primary care providers. (Legal; General Principles; Knowledge; Difficulty 2)

86. The answer is B. The lactation consultant is expected to communicate relevant information to the primary care provider(s). Referring her to another physician as the first strategy in helping her is inappropriate, although if she asks for the names of other providers, the LC should follow appropriate referral guidelines and provide these names. (Legal; 1 to 3 months; Knowledge; Difficulty 2)

87. The answer is C. The most effective protection against legal actions is establishing a mutually respectful relationship and rapport. (Legal; General Principles; Knowledge; Difficulty 4)

88. The answer is A. Each mother-baby system will develop unique feeding patterns. The LC supports any and all patterns that meet the mother and baby's needs. (Psychology; 1 to 2 days; Application; Difficulty 5)

89. The answer is A. Extreme nipple pain in the absence of visual symptoms may indicate a deeper problem such as prior history of abuse. (Psychology; 1 to 2 days; Knowledge; Difficulty 5)

90. The answer is D. All of the other items increase her empowerment. The "take-charge" attitude of the attendant puts her into a passive role, which has been shown to interfere with breastfeeding. (Psychology; Prenatal; Application; Difficulty 2)

91. The answer is A. Cultures that sexualize the breast are often the most resistant to women using their breasts to feed their infants anywhere and everywhere. (Psychology; General Principles; Knowledge; Difficulty 4)

92. The answer is D. Breastfeeding has little known effect on blood pressure. Any significant effect would likely to lower blood pressure because of the calming effects of lactational hormones. (Psychology; General Principles; Knowledge; Difficulty 2)

93. The answer is A. Support from her male partner is the most important of the options listed, although any support will increase the likelihood of her continuing to breastfeed. (Psychology; General Principles; Knowledge; Difficulty 4)

94. The answer is D. The oral experience of breastfeeding is pleasurable and normal. The infant controls and molds the shape of the breast in its mouth. (Psychology; General Principles; Application; Difficulty 2)

95. The answer is C. Fathers easily bond with their exclusively breastfed babies. (Psychology; 15 to 28 days; Application; Difficulty 3)

96. The answer is B. During the formal stage, mothers seek consistent, concrete "rules" to govern their actions. (Psychology; 3 to 14 days; Knowledge; Difficulty 4)

97. The answer is A. Exclusive breastfeeding is recommended for at least 6 months. Many babies show signs of readiness at that point, such as reaching for family foods. (Growth; 4 to 6 months; Application; Difficulty 3)

98. The answer is B. Lactogenesis II is triggered by the withdrawal of progesterone when the placenta separates. (Physiology; 1 to 2 days; Knowledge; Difficulty 4)

99. The answer is A. Her infant is probably experiencing a growth spurt. Initial breast edema is resolved, and the breasts are becoming "calibrated" to produce enough milk for her baby without feeding overful. (Growth; 1 to 3 months; Application; Difficulty 4)

100. The answer is D. This is a normal pattern on day 2. The baby's appetite, interest, and ability to feed will determine whether one or both breasts are taken at a given feeding. (Growth; 1 to 2 days; Application; Difficulty 5)

101. The answer is D. This is a period of equilibrium, and babies are more likely to wean in stable ages. (Growth; >12 months; Knowledge; Difficulty 4)

102. The answer is D. Scheduled feeds are inappropriate and can result in underfeeding and failure to thrive. The American Academy of Pediatrics and other experts advise feeding on cue regardless of the baby's age. (Growth; 1 to 3 months; Application; Difficulty 3)

103. The answer is B. The Baby-Friendly Hospital Initiative recommends that the baby breastfeed within the first 30 to 60 minutes after birth. (Growth; Labor/birth (perinatal); Application; Difficulty 4)

104. The answer is B. Babies start being able to self-feed around 6 months. (Growth; 4 to 6 months; Knowledge; Difficulty 4)

105. The answer is A. Breastfeeding the older child is mutually pleasurable even when the majority of the child's calories come from other sources. (Growth; >12 months; Knowledge; Difficulty 5)

106.   The answer is A. Forcing a baby to "cry it out" destroys the baby's growing sense of trust. Once broken, trust is difficult to repair. A baby's trust develops by consistently and promptly responding to her needs. Over time, her needs diminish and the baby can tolerate delays in mother's response. (Growth; 4 to 6 months; Application; Difficulty 2)

107.   The answer is C. Amount of milk pumped is the dependent variable. Use of the herb or a placebo is the independent variable. Weight gain of the babies is a confounding variable, since milk volume intake may not reflect actual milk volume produced. (Research; General Principles; Knowledge; Difficulty 3)

108.   The answer is B. Breastfed twins are often best friends and copy each other's breastfeeding behaviors. High milk volume may increase mother's susceptibility to milk stasis. (Growth; >12 months; Knowledge; Difficulty 3)

109.   The answer is B. Giving formula samples sends the message that the mother will need formula, thereby undermining breastfeeding. (Psychology; General Principles; Knowledge; Difficulty 2)

110.   The answer is D. Chickenpox is no longer contagious when all the lesions are completely crusted over. The mother can breastfeed normally. (Immunology; Labor/birth (perinatal); Application; Difficulty 5)

111.   The answer is B. Colostrum is rich in antiinfective and antiinflammatory properties. Its protective role appears to be even more important than its role in providing calories to the infant. (Immunology; 1 to 2 days; Knowledge; Difficulty 5)

112.   The answer is D. The length and/or frequency of breastfeeds are far less important causes of nipple damage than maternal skin conditions or the baby's ability to suck correctly. Most early cracked nipples are caused by poor breastfeeding technique and/or sucking problems. (Pathology; 1 to 2 days; Knowledge; Difficulty 5)

113.   The answer is D. The Babinski reflex, flaring of the toes, is triggered when the sole of the foot is stimulated. (Physiology; 1 to 2 days; Knowledge; Difficulty 4)

114.   The answer is D. WHO, UNICEF, and other authorities support providing the mother with confidential and individualized information to help her make a fully informed decision regarding feeding her baby. The lactation consultant's role is to assist the primary care physician and mother by providing appropriate research and other literature on the topic. (Legal; Prenatal; Application; Difficulty 5)

115.   The answer is C. All labor drugs cross the placenta, including those administered in the epidural space. The effect on the baby's ability to breastfeed appears to be dose-related. (Pharmacology; Labor/birth (perinatal); Application; Difficulty 5)

116. The answer is B. Operational definitions, or how the authors define the term *breastfeeding* is critical. (Research; General Principles; Application; Difficulty 3)

117. The answer is D. A research article published in a peer-reviewed professional journal is a primary reference. A is a review, which is a secondary reference. B is a chapter in a book, which is a secondary or tertiary source. C is a book, interpreting other sources in its recommendations. (Research; General Principles; Application; Difficulty 4)

118. The answer is B. Taking a thorough history is top priority when solving a breastfeeding problem. It is highly likely that the baby is having an allergic reaction to the large amount of milk consumed by the mother. (Techniques; General Principles; Application; Difficulty 3)

119. The answer is A. In order for a maternal medication to affect the baby, it must pass into milk and be ingested by the baby. Drugs that are not absorbed from the GI tract are very low risk because the baby's GI tract would not absorb the drug even if it's in the milk. (Pharmacology; General Principles; Knowledge; Difficulty 5)

120. The answer is A. The concentration of drug in the milk is nearly always proportional to the level in the maternal plasma. (Pharmacology; General Principles; Knowledge; Difficulty 2)

121. The answer is D. She had a bacterial infection of the nipple skin, most likely streptococcus transferred from the baby's mouth. The rash is exactly where the baby's mouth had come in contact with the areolar tissue. (Immunology; 4 to 6 months; Application; Difficulty 5)

122. The answer is D. This mother's breasts are entirely normal. Dripping milk is from duct openings is unlikely to have any affect on the baby's latch. Areolar size is unrelated to milk supply and ability to breastfeed. (Physiology; 3 to 14 days; Application; Difficulty 3)

123. The answer is C. The baby's mouth is infected with thrush (candida), which is a fungus. Mother and baby need to be treated simultaneously with an antifungal agent. (Pathology; 3 to 14 days; Application; Difficulty 5)

124. The answer is D. There is no research or epidemiological evidence that unrestricted breastfeeding at night is a cause of baby-bottle tooth decay or "nursing caries." The other choices are associated with rampant caries in young children. (Pathology; >12 months; Application; Difficulty 3)

125. The answer is C. This baby has Down syndrome. However, not all babies with Down syndrome have problems with breastfeeding. (Pathology; 15 to 28 days; Application; Difficulty 3)

126. The answer is D. The reddened areola and nipple area indicate the probable presence of nipple thrush (candida) infection, which is commonly accompanied by burning, stinging, or itching. Fever and chills and/or deep, aching breast pain are more likely to be caused by a bacterial breast infection. A few mothers will feel no discomfort even with this amount of nipple thrush. (Pathology; 15 to 28 days; Application; Difficulty 3)

127. The answer is B. The damage shown is infectious in origin, not mechanical. (Pathology; >12 months; Application; Difficulty 4)

128. The answer is A. Weaning from the affected breast following abscess formation or treatment is rarely necessary. All the other actions are appropriate. (Pathology; 1 to 3 months; Application; Difficulty 2)

129. The answer is D. This is a bacterial infection of the nipple skin. The baby had just begun treatment for a staph infection on its mouth that was acquired at day care. (Pathology; 15 to 28 days; Application; Difficulty 4)

130. The answer is A. The flattened nipple is MOST LIKELY causing a pinching nipple pain. This type of postfeed distortion is an indication that the baby did not feed well. (Pathology; 3 to 14 days; Application; Difficulty 4)

131. The answer is B. This mother's large, fibrous nipple was being compressed by her baby's small mouth and shallow palate. (Pathology; 3 to 14 days; Application; Difficulty 2)

132. The answer is C. Dressings designed for moist wound healing are appropriate treatments for nipple wounds. The source of the damage needs to be identified and corrected. The other suggestions are inappropriate. (Pathology; 15 to 28 days; Application; Difficulty 2)

133. The answer is A. This mother's breast has no visible areola. She experienced no breast changes during pregnancy, and this breast did not produce any milk postbirth. Sometimes one unusual finding, such as the lack of pigmented areola, indicates other unusual or pathological conditions. (Pathology; 3 to 14 days; Knowledge; Difficulty 3)

134. The answer is C. Emergency action is not warranted for this baby as there are no obvious indications of a life-threatening condition. The baby is slightly yellow (jaundiced) and sleepy, so the other choices are appropriate. (Pathology; 3 to 14 days; Application; Difficulty 2)

135. The answer is B. This mother has axillary mammary tissue which has no outlet, and the photo was taken 4 days postbirth. Lactogenesis II is causing milk secretion in the axillary mammary tissue. (Pathology; 3 to 14 days; Knowledge; Difficulty 3)

136. The answer is D. Supine sleeping is the safest position for sleeping. This position is next best, especially if the mother is sleeping next to the child. There is no published risk of being near an unused fireplace. Giving a pacifier may slightly reduce risk if a pacifier was used daily from birth. (Pathology; 15 to 28 days; Application; Difficulty 4)

137. The answer is B. The highest risk for SIDS is 2 to 4 months of age; the baby pictured is 3 months old. (Pathology; 1 to 3 months; Application; Difficulty 5)

138. The answer is B. The most likely cause of her nipple pain is off-center placement of the nipple in the pump flange. At one time, this was thought to increase milk yield. (Pathology; 3 to 14 days; Application; Difficulty 4)

139. The answer is B. Fungal infections on the lactating breast are typically not localized to one small area. The other conditions are more likely, and the lactation consultant should be collaborating with her medical care provider for a thorough diagnosis. (Pathology; 4 to 6 months; Knowledge; Difficulty 3)

140. The answer is C. This is an entirely normal breast with moderate fullness. There are no visual indications of mastitis, galactocele, or edema. (Physiology; 15 to 28 days; Knowledge; Difficulty 5)

141. The answer is C. This mother's breasts are full and taut with milk, which inhibits her baby from a good deep latch. She should express or pump some milk to soften her breasts before trying to feed him again. (Pathology; 3 to 14 days; Application; Difficulty 3)

142. The answer is C. Immediate skin-to-skin contact is an excellent strategy to calm and warm a baby in preparation for breastfeeding. (Physiology; 1 to 2 days; Application; Difficulty 4)

143. The answer is B. This baby is in the quiet alert state. (Physiology; 15 to 28 days; Knowledge; Difficulty 4)

144. The answer is D. This mother still had bright red vaginal bleeding and a very low milk supply. This situation strongly suggests a retained placenta, which suppresses the onset of lactogenesis II. (Physiology; 3 to 14 days; Application; Difficulty 4)

145. The answer is A. The peaked shape with barely visible damage in the center of the nipple tip is most often associated with either a poor (shallow) latch, or a baby with a sucking problem. In this case, the baby was tongue-tied. Rarely would a deeply latched baby cause this severe nipple distortion. When a baby is poorly latched or has a suck deficit, effective milk transfer and self-detachment are less likely. (Techniques; 1 to 2 days; Application; Difficulty 4)

146. The answer is D. Many, if not most, babies sleep better when close to their mothers or carried on their mothers' bodies. This is normal behavior. (Growth; 4 to 6 months; Knowledge; Difficulty 2)

147. The answer is C. This 4-week-old baby has gained weight rapidly and is entirely normal. (Physiology; 15 to 28 days; Knowledge; Difficulty 3)

148. The answer is A. Slight differences in breast size during lactation are normal and common. (Anatomy; 15 to 28 days; Application; Difficulty 2)

149. The answer is C. This baby's lingual frenulum, the string-like tissue between the tongue and the floor of the mouth, is short and tight and likely to restrict tongue motion needed for effective feeding. (Anatomy; 1 to 2 days; Application; Difficulty 3)

150. The answer is A. This child is tongue-tied, often referred to as ankyloglossia. The lingual frenulum is short and/or tight. Without full normal tongue mobility, breastfeeding and eating (and other activities involving movement of the tongue) are compromised. (Anatomy; >12 months; Knowledge; Difficulty 3)

151. The answer is B. This nipple is flat. There is no distinct "shank" between the areola and nipple "bud" or tip. (Anatomy; 15 to 28 days; Knowledge; Difficulty 4)

152. The answer is D. This mother's nipple size is in the normal range, therefore this answer is incorrect. A, B, and C are true statements; the breast and nipple are entirely normal. The puckering around the areola is probably because the air is cool. Her areola diameter is on the narrow end of normal diameter. (Anatomy; Preconception; Application; Difficulty 2)

153. The answer is B. The small breast has characteristics of insufficient glandular tissue. (Anatomy; 15 to 28 days; Application; Difficulty 4)

154. The answer is C. The raised areas on her areola are normal Montgomery glands. This is a normal breast. (Anatomy; >12 months; Application; Difficulty 2)

155. The answer is D. This is a normal breast. (Anatomy; Prenatal; Application; Difficulty 4)

156. The answer is D. Hypermastia, or accessory mammary tissue, may be found along the "milk lines," which run from the upper inner arm to the inguinal region. Accessory mammary tissue develops during fetal development. (Anatomy; 3 to 14 days; Application; Difficulty 4)

157. The answer is B. Milk collected during mastitis does not contain pus, and there is no indication that the mother has a breast infection. Yellow color milk can be caused by A, C, and D. On day 5, C is most likely the cause of the yellow color in this milk sample. (Pharmacology; 3 to 14 days; Application; Difficulty 2)

158. The answer is B. This is an allergic rash that began when the baby ingested cow's milk–based infant formula at day care. (Immunology; 7 to 12 months; Application; Difficulty 5)

159. The answer is B. This eczema, an allergic reaction that began soon after this baby was given supplements of cow milk–based formula. Rice cereal is a less common allergen. It is unlikely that cold temperature or a tetanus immunization triggered this response. (Immunology; 15 to 28 days; Application; Difficulty 3)

160. The answer is C. The average 2- to 4-week-old baby's milk consumption is 750 ml (25 oz) per day. The amount can vary widely among normal babies. (Biochemistry; 15 to 28 days; Application; Difficulty 5)

161. The answer is C. Fats in milk do not increase over time. All of the other components increase as lactation progresses over time. (Biochemistry; 7 to 12 months; Knowledge; Difficulty 3)

162. The answer is B. The indentation visible on the areolar skin was caused by a breast shell placed over her nipple to allow air drying of the wound. (Equipment; 3 to 14 days; Application; Difficulty 4)

163. The answer is A. On day 4, many mothers make more milk than their infants can consume. Use of a pump to remove excess milk can help prevent milk stasis and help the baby latch on and feed more effectively. (Equipment; 3 to 14 days; Application; Difficulty 5)

164. The answer is C. Cup-feeding may not necessarily prevent nipple confusion. The other answers are correct. (Equipment; 3 to 14 days; Application; Difficulty 2)

165. The answer is D. Using a nipple shield is unlikely to reduce cross-infection, and a child of this age will likely vigorously object to introduction of this device. (Equipment; 4 to 6 months; Application; Difficulty 2)

166. The answer is C. Assuring proper positioning and latch is always the first action. This mother's bifurcated nipple was fully functional, and the baby fed from this breast easily and effectively. (Techniques; 3 to 14 days; Application; Difficulty 4)

167. The answer is C. This baby is adequately attached and positioned for feeding, and the pattern is normal in length and comfortable for both mother and baby. While A, B, and D would be appropriate if the feeding pattern was uncomfortable or ineffective, suggesting too many technique changes could undermine the mother's confidence in breastfeeding. (Techniques; 15 to 28 days; Application; Difficulty 2)

168. The answer is D. Finger-feeding is a therapeutic method to help a baby get back to direct breastfeeding. After palate repair, a soft object (like a breast) is less likely to hurt or damage the repair site. (Techniques; 15 to 28 days; Application; Difficulty 3)

169. The answer is B. This mother's breast is engorged—a combination of edema and milk stasis. Hot compresses can make edema worse and have no documented advantage in correcting milk stasis. (Techniques; 3 to 14 days; Application; Difficulty 5)

170. The answer is B. The baby's lower lip is curled in and needs to be turned (flanged) outward. Tickling the baby's feet is ineffective, and there is no need to press down on the breast to clear his nostrils. (Techniques; 3 to 14 days; Application; Difficulty 4)

171. The answer is A. The vertical position is helpful when the baby has a head injury or needs help maintaining good alignment. Let-down reflex is not affected by baby's position; the "colic hold" is holding the baby prone on the mother's forearm. Plugged milk ducts are rarely found in the upper quadrant. (Techniques; 15 to 28 days; Application; Difficulty 2)

172. The answer is C. Wound cleaning is not a standard part of lactation consultant practice. The other actions are appropriate. (Techniques; 1 to 3 months; Application; Difficulty 3)

173. The answer is A. This baby's diaper-area rash was caused by candida (thrush) infection, which was also present in his mouth and on mother's nipples. Mother was experiencing itching, stinging, burning nipple pain consistent with thrush infection of the nipples. (Pathology; 15 to 28 days; Application; Difficulty 4)

174. The answer is C. This 9-month-old baby may self-feed with a pincer grasp, sip liquids from an open cup, and/or breastfeed 8 to 16 times a day or as often as a newborn. It is highly unlikely that she would self-wean at this age. (Techniques; 7 to 12 months; Application; Difficulty 3)

175. The answer is B. A clear description of your observation is most appropriate. Option A is less clear; C is offering a diagnosis, and D includes the mother's subjective feelings ("painful"). (Techniques; General Principles; Application; Difficulty 5)

176. The answer is C. Finger-feeding is one appropriate technique for improving a baby's suboptimum suck, providing food, allowing nipples to heal, and behavior modification. (Techniques; 3 to 14 days; Application; Difficulty 4)

177. The answer is B. The hand is pinching the base of the nipple, cutting off milk flow. This could also bruise the areola, and there is no published evidence that nipple rolling will improve nipple elasticity. (Techniques; >12 months; Application; Difficulty 4)

178. The answer is C. This baby's most immediate need is for calories. His skin is slightly yellow, suggesting some amount of jaundice. That fact, combined with 2 weeks of poor feeding at breast, indicates inadequate milk transfer. The baby needs calories immediately while other approaches to remedy this situation are explored. (Techniques; 3 to 14 days; Application; Difficulty 5)

179. The answer is A. Always evaluate the baby's breastfeeding technique first. This mother's baby was tongue-tied, and friction from his tongue was causing the persistent nipple wound. (Techniques; 1 to 3 months; Application; Difficulty 4)

180. The answer is C. She is attempting to pull the nipple tip outward. (Techniques; Prenatal; Application; Difficulty 2)

181. The answer is A. This mother is gently and correctly rolling her retracted nipples to firm them prior to feeding. (Techniques; 1 to 2 days; Application; Difficulty 4)

182. The answer is C. This technique is ineffective for expressing milk, but might be helpful for the other situations listed. (Techniques; 1 to 2 days; Knowledge; Difficulty 4)

183. The answer is A. Large breasts often need to be supported while the baby feeds. This mother's breast is large, but there is no evidence of milk stasis, edema, or excessive fullness. (Techniques; 3 to 14 days; Application; Difficulty 3)

184. The answer is B. Baby Bs rate of weight gain was the fastest, as represented by the steeply increasing angle of slope of the graph. None of the other conclusions can be drawn from the data presented. (Research; 15 to 28 days; Application; Difficulty 3)

185. The answer is C. Breastfeeding with complementary family foods is recommended by UNICEF and the World Health Organization for the child in her second 6 months of life. (Public Health; 7 to 12 months; Knowledge; Difficulty 4)

186. The answer is B. Young children imitating breastfeeding with a doll is a common and normal occurrence in most cultures worldwide. (Psychology; Preconception; Application; Difficulty 2)

187. The answer is D. Siblings sleeping together is a practice found in many cultures. There is no evidence that siblings napping together puts either child in danger. (Psychology; 15 to 28 days; Application; Difficulty 4)

188. The answer is D. The LC should help the mother clarify her feelings about continuing to breastfeed, and support her decision. The other responses are not appropriate. (Psychology; Prenatal; Application; Difficulty 3)

189. The answer is C. It is always appropriate to begin a counseling session with an open-ended, general, supportive question. Option B is inappropriate at 2 months, the age of the baby pictured. A would be a reasonable question, especially if nipple soreness is a problem. D might be asked on a routine screening form. (Psychology; 1 to 3 months; Application; Difficulty 4)

190. The answer is A. Mothers of multiples often attach to the "unit" before the individual baby or babies. (Psychology; 7 to 12 months; Knowledge; Difficulty 3)

191. The answer is C. This is least likely to be an abscess because there is no redness or discoloration. The bulge on this woman's areola at the 10:00 position was a galactocele and caused her no discomfort or difficulty breastfeeding. (Pathology; 1 to 2 days; Knowledge; Difficulty 5)

192. The answer is C. Persistent biting is not common in nursing toddlers. Any attempts at biting should be immediately stopped by mother. (Growth; >12 months; Application; Difficulty 3)

193. The answer is C. The 2 to 4 week old is not yet capable of reaching for objects. (Growth; 15 to 28 days; Application; Difficulty 2)

194. The answer is A. This child is obviously thriving—his growth is not faltering in the slightest. Avoidance of certain foods, including common family foods, appears to be not unusual in babies from allergic families. (Growth; 4 to 6 months; Application; Difficulty 4)

195. The answer is B. Appropriate exclusive breastfeeding is unlikely to cause this pattern. The other conditions could result in growth compromise as charted. (Growth; 7 to 12 months; Knowledge; Difficulty 5)

196. The answer is B. "Gymnastic" nursing, pincer grasp and self-feeding, and increased mobility are typical of the 7- to 12-month-old baby. (Growth; 7 to 12 months; Knowledge; Difficulty 5)

197. The answer is B. There is no research evidence of increased risk to the baby from a sober, nonsmoking mother. A, B, and D are well-documented benefits of breastfeeding at night. (Growth; 1 to 3 months; Application; Difficulty 2)

198. The answer is D. Pre-2000 growth curves published by the National Center for Health Statistics were not based on exclusively breastfed babies. Newer research has established that artificially fed babies are fatter (heavier) per length compared with breastfed babies in the 3 to 6 month period. The baby pictured is 4 months old. (Growth; 4 to 6 months; Application; Difficulty 4)

199. The answer is C. Separation anxiety is very common around 8 months, the age of the child pictured. (Growth; 7 to 12 months; Application; Difficulty 3)

200. The answer is C. The tongue extrusion reflex fades (integrates) by 6 months. The child shown is $8^{1}/_{2}$ months old. Stepping at this age is not a reflex, but a deliberate behavior. (Growth; 7 to 12 months; Knowledge; Difficulty 5)

EXAM C

1. The answer is A. Magnesium sulfate can cause maternal drowsiness and lethargy. The American Academy of Pediatrics considers this medication compatible with breastfeeding. (Pharmacology; 1 to 2 days; Knowledge; Difficulty 5)

2. The answer is C. Herbs can pass into milk and exert an effect on the baby. Giving pharmaceutical advice is not within the scope of practice of the lactation consultant. (Pharmacology; General Principles; Application; Difficulty 2)

3. The answer is B. Epidural analgesia and narcotics cross the placenta and have documented effects on the baby's motor and neurobehavioral scores. (Pharmacology; Labor/birth (perinatal); Application; Difficulty 2)

4. The answer is C. About 1% of most medications given to a lactating woman actually gets to her breastfed baby. (Pharmacology; General Principles; Knowledge; Difficulty 3)

5. The answer is B. Drugs more readily pass into milk in the first few days postbirth because the junctures between mammary secretory cells are open at this point, permitting passage of medications and other substances into the alveolar lumen. (Pharmacology; 1 to 2 days; Knowledge; Difficulty 3)

6. The answer is C. Caffeine is the most likely to affect the baby because it is a CNS stimulant and highly lipid soluble. Insulin is poorly absorbed orally; digoxin acts on muscle tissue and passes poorly into milk; warfarin has a large molecular weight and does not pass into milk. (Pharmacology; General Principles; Application; Difficulty 2)

7. The answer is C. There are a myriad of potential breastfeeding problems associated with epidural anesthesia. (Pharmacology; Labor/birth (perinatal); Application; Difficulty 2)

8. The answer is C. After 5 half-lives have passed, approximately 98% of the drug or isotope have been eliminated. Each drug or isotope has a specific half-life. (Pharmacology; General Principles; Knowledge; Difficulty 3)

9. The answer is C. Homeopathic remedies have the least effect. Homeopathic remedies are extremely dilute preparations. (Pharmacology; 15 to 28 days; Knowledge; Difficulty 4)

10. The answer is B. Babies are not lazy. Labeling babies in this manner prevents looking for, finding, and resolving the cause of the problem. (Pathology; 15 to 28 days; Application; Difficulty 5)

11. The answer is A. It is always appropriate to make sure the baby is feeding well as the FIRST strategy. While that level of bilirubin is rarely a problem for a healthy, fullterm newborn, the LC should always make sure the baby is effectively feeding as a top priority. (Pathology; 3 to 14 days; Application; Difficulty 3)

12. The answer is D. Mothers with hearing impairments are very familiar with visual and tactile communication. Breastfeeding may be easier for her than artificial feeding. (Pathology; 1 to 2 days; Application; Difficulty 4)

13. The answer is D. Mammary duct ectasia is the most likely cause of nipple discharge in early lactation. The other conditions do not cause greenish discharge. (Pathology; 1 to 2 days; Knowledge; Difficulty 4)

14. The answer is B. Maternal diabetes increases the risk of breast infections. (Pathology; 15 to 28 days; Knowledge; Difficulty 2)

15. The answer is A. Lactose promotes the absorption of iron. Lactoferrin indirectly helps establish intestinal flora, by keeping the pathogenic population in check, but it does not directly promote the growth of beneficial bacteria in the gut. (Pathology; 3 to 14 days; Knowledge; Difficulty 5)

16. The answer is C. When standard, appropriate treatment for breast engorgement do not quickly resolve the problem, a thorough medical evaluation is warranted to confirm or rule out serious pathology. (Pathology; 3 to 14 days; Application; Difficulty 3)

17. The answer is C. The most likely explanation for this infant's behavior is overactive milk ejection reflex. (Physiology; 3 to 14 days; Application; Difficulty 3)

18. The answer is C. Babies feed for varying lengths and at varying intervals according to their hunger, emotional needs, growth and developmental stages, and other physiological factors. Placing restrictions on length or frequency, or offering "substitutes" disrupts the breastfeeding relationship and interferes with fulfillment of infant needs. (Physiology; 15 to 28 days; Application; Difficulty 2)

19. The answer is D. Most mothers will produce plenty of milk for several breastfed babies, despite higher risk of early birth-related problems. (Physiology; 15 to 28 days; Knowledge; Difficulty 2)

20. The answer is C. The timing of lactogenesis II is not affected by the mode/route of delivery. (Physiology; Labor/birth (perinatal); Knowledge; Difficulty 3)

21. The answer is C. Allowing the baby to finish the first breast first allows the baby's appetite to best determine the balance of nutrients he obtains during a feed. Enforcing other patterns may result in less than optimal intake of nutrients and calories. (Physiology; 1 to 2 days; Application; Difficulty 5)

22. The answer is D. Lactation Amenorrhea Method is the most compatible with breastfeeding. Condoms are also a first choice but less reliable. Progestin-only methods are second choices, and methods containing estrogen are third choices. (Physiology; 4 to 6 months; Knowledge; Difficulty 4)

23. The answer is B. Thorough removal milk will increase the RATE of milk synthesis. Stimulation without removal is not effective because milk stasis slows the rate of milk synthesis. Galactagogues are not well researched. Metaclopromide will increase prolactin, but needs to be combined with adequate milk removal. (Physiology; 3 to 14 days; Application; Difficulty 5)

24. The answer is B. Babies typically take 75% to 85% of the available milk during any given feeding. (Physiology; 15 to 28 days; Application; Difficulty 3)

25. The answer is C. Small breasts usually have less storage capacity than larger breasts, so frequent expression triggers a high rate of milk synthesis. The rate of synthesis is fastest when the breasts are "emptiest", so expressing until the flow ceases will also maximize the rate of milk synthesis. (Physiology; Prematurity; Application; Difficulty 4)

26. The answer is D. Hearing and taste develop early in gestation. All the other processes are compromised by preterm birth. (Physiology; Prematurity; Knowledge; Difficulty 2)

27. The answer is D. The alveoli are positioned back in the breast tissue, and rarely are inside the baby's mouth. A portion of the areola should be inside the infant's mouth, but not necessarily all of it, depending on the areola diameter. A portion of the lactiferous sinuses will be inside the baby's mouth. (Anatomy; 1 to 2 days; Application; Difficulty 2)

28. The answer is B. The Montgomery glands are sebaceous glands which produce oil to lubricate the nipple and areolar skin, and may have other functions. (Anatomy; General Principles; Application; Difficulty 4)

29. The answer is D. Artificially fed children are more likely to need orthodontia, have weakened masseter muscles, and more speech disorders. (Anatomy; >12 months; Knowledge; Difficulty 5)

30. The answer is C. Severing nerve pathways would be the worst consequence to lactation. (Anatomy; Preconception; Application; Difficulty 5)

31. The answer is B. The tongue usually extends past the lower gum ridge (alveolar ridge) and is cupped around the breast. Occasionally, it will extend past the lower lip. (Anatomy; General Principles; Application; Difficulty 4)

32. The answer is A. Reflux may be caused by an esophageal defect at the upper sphincter, where the esophagus meets the stomach. (Anatomy; Prenatal; Application; Difficulty 2)

33. The answer is C. The alveoli contain secretory cells which produce milk. (Anatomy; General Principles; Knowledge; Difficulty 3)

34. The answer is B. Ovarian function postbirth is not related to lactation. The other statements are relevant. (Anatomy; Labor/birth (perinatal); Application; Difficulty 2)

35. The answer is B. The hypoglossal nerve is the primary motor nerve of the tongue, therefore an inability to move the tongue to compress the breast is the most likely result of damage to this nerve. (Anatomy; Labor/birth (perinatal); Application; Difficulty 5)

36. The answer is B. Placing the fingers at the edge of the areola is the best place to begin assessing a nipple-areola complex for inversion. (Anatomy; Prenatal; Application; Difficulty 5)

37. The answer is C. There is no evidence that the mother will become less ill because she is lactating. Antibodies and white cells that she produces quickly get into her milk and protect the baby, and a mother who is sick certainly does not benefit from the additional work of preparing artificial feeds and coping with probable sudden milk stasis. (Immunology; 4 to 6 months; Application; Difficulty 2)

38. The answer is D. Although sudden, severe latex allergies are possible, the reaction is more likely to be caused by an ingested allergen, especially cow's milk protein. All of the other choices are possible routes of sensitization. (Immunology; 15 to 28 days; Application; Difficulty 2)

39. The answer is C. No studies have yet reported on a direct correlation between CHD and infant feeding, although recent studies of adolescents show an increase in serum lipids in those who were artificially fed. A significant relationship to mode of infant feeding has been shown in the other conditions. (Immunology; Preconception; Knowledge; Difficulty 5)

40. The answer is A. To date, studies have not established a relationship between gross motor performance and infant feeding mode. The other elements are strongly linked to duration and intensity of breastfeeding. (Immunology; General Principles; Knowledge; Difficulty 5)

41. The answer is A. Complement is a biochemical pathway for inflammation and is poorly represented in human milk. (Immunology; 12, General Principles; Knowledge; Difficulty 5)

42. The answer is B. Mother's milk helps build baby's immune system. Environmental chemicals that may appear in mother's milk have no documented effect on the baby or its immune system. (Immunology; General Principles; Knowledge; Difficulty 2)

43. The answer is D. White cells in milk do not directly attack dietary allergens. The other answers are true. (Immunology; General Principles; Knowledge; Difficulty 2)

44. The answer is B. Allergic reactions to fortifiers based on bovine milk are a serious problem for preterm babies. (Immunology; Prematurity; Knowledge; Difficulty 2)

45. The answer is C. Estrogen in human milk does not appear to have an immunologic function. (Biochemistry; General Principles; Knowledge; Difficulty 5)

46. The answer is C. Lactose levels are constant and stable at all times except the colostral phase, when lactose is low. (Biochemistry; General Principles; Knowledge; Difficulty 4)

47. The answer is D. Research in Australia has found that the relative fullness of the breast accounts for 70% of the fat variation in milk. (Biochemistry; General Principles; Knowledge; Difficulty 4)

48. The answer is D. Trigylcerides are the predominant lipids in human milk. (Biochemistry; General Principles; Knowledge; Difficulty 5)

49. The answer is B. Vitamins B6 and B12 in milk are strongly dependent on maternal dietary intake. These nutrients are essential to the baby. (Biochemistry; General Principles; Knowledge; Difficulty 2)

50. The answer is D. Most breastfeeding mothers can follow the eating and fluid intake patterns of an average woman in the United States. (Biochemistry; General Principles; Knowledge; Difficulty 4)

51. The answer is B. Colostrum has 2 to 3 g/100 ml, mature milk has 4 to 5 g/100 ml of fat. (Biochemistry; 1 to 2 days; Knowledge; Difficulty 3)

52. The answer is D. WHO recommends other foods in the opposite order of priority. (Biochemistry; General Principles; Knowledge; Difficulty 4)

53. The answer is A. Omega-3 fatty acids DHA and AA are especially important in development of the central nervous system and are found in abundance in human milk. (Biochemistry; General Principles; Knowledge; Difficulty 3)

54. The answer is D. Adding iron to the breastfed baby's diet may increase risk of illness by overwhelming the lactoferrin. (Biochemistry; General Principles; Knowledge; Difficulty 2)

55. The answer is A. A well-balanced diet with adequate calories is important for the mother's overall health. Most milk components are not substantially related to mother's dietary intake. (Biochemistry; Prenatal; Application; Difficulty 4)

56. The answer is D. Pasteurized donor milk from screened donors does not transmit the HIV virus. Pasteurization kills the virus. (Biochemistry; General Principles; Knowledge; Difficulty 2)

57. The answer is A. Lactoferrin binds to iron, which starves pathogenic bacteria of the iron needed to proliferate. (Biochemistry; General Principles; Knowledge; Difficulty 5)

58. The answer is B. On days 1 to 3, the baby gets about 30 ml/day of colostrum. As lactogenesis II occurs, baby obtains more per day as milk volume rapidly rises to about 600 ml/day or more by day 5. (Biochemistry; 1 to 2 days; Knowledge; Difficulty 4)

59. The answer is C. Lactoferrin binds iron in milk and makes it available to the infant. Adding additional sources of dietary iron overwhelms the lactoferrin, leaving the iron available to pathogenic bacteria for growth. (Biochemistry; 4 to 6 months; Knowledge; Difficulty 4)

60. The answer is C. Lysozyme is stable at temperatures used for pasteurization. All of the other properties are true. (Biochemistry; Prematurity; Knowledge; Difficulty 2)

61. The answer is D. Mothers' dietary practices have very little effect on lactation. Following good dietary practices is important for the breastfeeding mother's general health. (Biochemistry; General Principles; Application; Difficulty 5)

62. The answer is A. Pacifiers are alleged to improve dentition, but research supports more orthodontic problems in children who use pacifiers. (Equipment; 15 to 28 days; Knowledge; Difficulty 2)

63. The answer is C. Pumps should operate at about the same number of cycles per minutes, as the baby would feed: 40 to 60 times per minute. (Equipment; General Principles; Knowledge; Difficulty 3)

64. The answer is C. Prolactin levels are unaffected by thin silicone nipple shields. (Equipment; 3 to 14 days; Knowledge; Difficulty 5)

65. The answer is D. Glass is the recommended storage container for mother's own milk. Hard plastic (polycarbonate or polypropylene) containers with lids are acceptable. (Equipment; Prematurity; Knowledge; Difficulty 2)

66. The answer is C. A thin silicone nipple shield is fairly easy to keep clean and should be cleaned thoroughly after each use. However, the risk of contamination by pathogens is still present. The other risks listed are more significant. (Equipment; 3 to 14 days; Application; Difficulty 5)

67. The answer is C. Cold packs will reduce edema, the most likely cause of impeded milk flow in early postpartum. There is no research supporting the use of hot compresses to improve milk flow. (Equipment; 3 to 14 days; Application; Difficulty 3)

68. The answer is D. Using a supplementer at breast to increase milk volume is only effective when the baby's suck is effective. (Techniques; 1 to 2 days; Application; Difficulty 5)

69. The answer is C. The mother is experiencing milk stasis and inflammation, a common event on day 3. Removal of milk and control of edema are top priorities. (Techniques; 3 to 14 days; Application; Difficulty 2)

70. The answer is C. Skin-to-skin contact helps babies initiate breast-feeding. (Techniques; 1 to 2 days; Application; Difficulty 3)

71. The answer is B. Sucking on fists is a feeding cue, which should be responded to by offering the breast. (Techniques; Prematurity; Application; Difficulty 2)

72. The answer is B. Macrophages and possibly neutrophils and T-lymphocytes actively kill microbes by phagocytosis. (Techniques; 1 to 2 days; Knowledge; Difficulty 4)

73. The answer is A. Exclusive breastfeeding means that the baby satisfies all nutrition and sucking at his mother's breast. Option B has use of devices; Option C includes other fluids, and Option D could include other fluids and/or pacifiers. (Research; General Principles; Knowledge; Difficulty 5)

74. The answer is B. Randomized controlled trials are considered the most rigorous evidence for a phenomenon. (Research; General Principles; Knowledge; Difficulty 3)

75. The answer is B. False negative (type II) errors occur when a real difference exists, but a flaw in the design or other aspect of the research does not identify the real difference. Inadequate sample size is one cause of type II errors. Choice A is a type I error, and a control group is necessary for any comparative analysis of groups. (Research; General Principles; Knowledge; Difficulty 3)

76. The answer is B. Operational definitions, or how the authors define the term *breastfeeding* is critical. (Research; General Principles; Application; Difficulty 3)

77. The answer is B. World Breastfeeding Week themes focus on benefits of breastfeeding and positive changes to facilitate breastfeeding. Forcing mothers to breastfeed is inappropriate. (Public Health; General Principles; Knowledge; Difficulty 2)

78. The answer is B. The Code specifies that information on artificial feeding provided to health workers should be scientific and accurate. Detailed accurate information on product composition is appropriate marketing of products within the scope of the Code. (Public Health; General Principles; Knowledge; Difficulty 2)

79. The answer is B. Preterm milk is higher in protein, sodium, and chloride. (Biochemistry; Prematurity; Knowledge; Difficulty 3)

80. The answer is C. The Baby Friendly Hospital Initiative is designed to protect breastfed babies from practices and policies that disrupt or interfere with breastfeeding. (Public Health; 1 to 2 days; Knowledge; Difficulty 4)

81. The answer is B. Child survival programs advocate exclusive breastfeeding as the best nutrition for the first 6 months, and breastfeeding as an excellent staple food for up to 2 years or more. (Public Health; General Principles; Knowledge; Difficulty 3)

82. The answer is C. The mother should breastfeed her baby within a half-hour of birth. Newer research indicates that most babies will begin breastfeeding within the first hour if left undisturbed on mother's chest/abdomen following birth. (Public Health; Labor/birth (perinatal); Knowledge; Difficulty 4)

83. The answer is D. The lactation consultant may be asked to serve as an expert witness in divorce and custody situations involving a breastfed baby or lactating mother. The LC should always assist the mother in maintaining an intact breastfeeding relationship with her child. (Legal; General Principles; Application; Difficulty 2)

84. The answer is A. Communicating relevant information to primary care provider(s) is required of lactation consultants. (Legal; General Principles; Application; Difficulty 3)

85. The answer is C. Original research (primary references) is the most important type of source to include in a literature review. Texts and review articles may help you locate primary references on a subject. Lectures also may direct you to primary references. (Research; General Principles; Application; Difficulty 4)

86. The answer is A. Consent must be obtained before touching the mother or baby or taking photographs. Unwanted touching could be considered battery. Written consent is preferred over verbal. (Legal; General Principles; Knowledge; Difficulty 2)

87. The answer is D. Telling others of her pregnancy is an early developmental task. Failure to reveal her pregnancy suggests lack of acceptance of the fetus. (Psychology; Prenatal; Knowledge; Difficulty 2)

88. The answer is D. The other areas may have extra mammary and/or nipple tissue, which are remnants of the galactic band. (Anatomy; Preconception; Knowledge; Difficulty 3)

89. The answer is B. Research shows mothers rest better when mothers and babies are kept together following birth. (Psychology; Labor/birth (perinatal); Knowledge; Difficulty 2)

90. The answer is C. While partial breastfeeding is better than none, the other options should be pursued first. (Psychology; General Principles; Knowledge; Difficulty 5)

91. The answer is A. Separate sleeping is a recent and unusual developmental pattern for babies. (Psychology; 7 to 12 months; Knowledge; Difficulty 5)

92. The answer is D. Facilitating continued direct breastfeeding is better for the breastfeeding relationship. However, even just having facilities for collecting milk is a positive support for breastfeeding. (Psychology; General Principles; Knowledge; Difficulty 2)

93. The answer is A. The mother's age is only somewhat significant to her experience. Other societal factors appear to have more a powerful affect on her comfort or discomfort with her maternal role. (Psychology; Labor/birth (perinatal); Knowledge; Difficulty 2)

94. The answer is B is the most supportive statement because it is an open-ended question designed to explore the mother's preconceived ideas about breastfeeding. (Psychology; Prenatal; Application; Difficulty 3)

95. The answer is C. The breastfeeding dyad is a unique biological and psychological entity. (Psychology; General Principles; Knowledge; Difficulty 5)

96. The answer is D. Medications to relieve labor pain can significantly interfere with breastfeeding and bonding. The other elements of the plan enhance breastfeeding success. (Psychology; Labor/birth (perinatal); Application; Difficulty 2)

97. The answer is D. Experience and research show that 8 to 12 feeds totaling 140 to 160 minutes are most typical in industrialized cultures. Under 100 minutes at breast per day may indicate a problem. (Growth; 1 to 3 months; Application; Difficulty 4)

98. The answer is A. The older child is usually nursing for far more than food. Breastfeeding the older child is mutually pleasurable even when the majority of the child's calories come from other sources. (Growth; >12 months; Knowledge; Difficulty 2)

99. The answer is A. Forcing a baby to "cry it out" destroys the baby's growing sense of trust. Once broken, trust is difficult to repair. Babies' trust develops by consistently and promptly responding to his needs. Over time, his needs diminish and the baby can tolerate delays in mother's response. (Growth; 1 to 3 months; Application; Difficulty 2)

100. The answer is D. Nursing strikes are indications that the baby is having some difficulty with breastfeeding or the mother-baby breastfeeding relationship. Self-weaning before 12 months of age is unusual. (Growth; 7 to 12 months; Knowledge; Difficulty 2)

101. The answer is D. Anthropological evidence suggests the human infant was "designed" to breastfeed for more than 2 years. (Growth; >12 months; Knowledge; Difficulty 4)

102. The answer is B. There is no documented harm to either the fetus or older baby by continuing to breastfeed. Nipple pain during pregnancy is hormonally based and may be unavoidable. (Growth; Prenatal; Application; Difficulty 4)

103. The answer is A. Research and experience shows that a range of 7 to 30 minutes per breast is normal and common. (Growth; 15 to 28 days; Application; Difficulty 3)

104. The answer is B. There is no age beyond which breastfeeding is inappropriate. Complementary foods should begin some time in the second 6 months of life. (Growth; >12 months; Knowledge; Difficulty 4)

105. The answer is D. Most mothers will produce plenty of milk for several breastfed babies, despite higher risk of early birth-related problems. (Growth; 7 to 12 months; Application; Difficulty 3)

106. The answer is A. Epidural or anesthetic drugs cross the placenta and appear in cord blood. Epidurals are documented to increase the pushing stage of labor and increase the likelihood of operative birth. (Pharmacology; Labor/birth (perinatal); Application; Difficulty 2)

107. The answer is D. The foramen magnum is the large opening in the cranium (skull) through which passes the spinal cord. (Anatomy; Prenatal; Knowledge; Difficulty 2)

108. The answer is A. This is the biological norm, and most common nighttime arrangement worldwide. Separate sleeping is common in some Western cultures. Self-comforting may be distressful for some babies. Pacifiers can compromise breastfeeding. (Growth; 1 to 3 months; Application; Difficulty 3)

109. The answer is D. Normal babies without injury can nearly always feed in various positions on either breast. A baby who has sustained a birth injury may only have one position where breastfeeding is comfortable and successful. Over time as the injuries heal, he should be able to feed in a variety of positions. (Pathology; Labor/birth (perinatal); Knowledge; Difficulty 5)

110. The answer is D. Lack of eye contact and little talking to or caressing of her infant may be signs of postpartum depression. The LC should report these signs to the mother's primary care provider immediately. (Pathology; 1 to 2 days; Knowledge; Difficulty 4)

111. The answer is B. Low thyroid levels can cause suppressed milk synthesis, fatigue, and chilliness. The mother should have a full medical evaluation. (Pathology; 1 to 3 months; Knowledge; Difficulty 5)

112. The answer is B. Painful stimulation is not appropriate, and may even cause the baby to shut down further. (Techniques; 1 to 2 days; Application; Difficulty 3)

113. The answer is A. Hospitalization is usually a traumatic experience for the child, and the emotional comfort from breastfeeding is especially important at that time. (Techniques; 7 to 12 months; Application; Difficulty 2)

114. The answer is A. Antibiotic drugs have no documented affect on the fetus or newborn's ability to breastfeed. The other choices are more likely to contribute to breastfeeding difficulties. (Pharmacology; Labor/birth (perinatal); Application; Difficulty 2)

115. The answer is D. Case reports are the weakest form of evidence for a given policy or practice. Systematic reviews and meta-analyses are the strongest. (Research; General Principles; Knowledge; Difficulty 2)

116. The answer is A. Colostrum is the treatment of choice for asymptomatic hypoglycemia. A small amount of colostrum stabilizes blood sugar. Some methods of testing blood sugar are not accurate. Direct breastfeeding is always the first and best course of action. A newborn normally breastfeeds every 1 to 3 hours in the first 24 hours, and nothing in this question indicates when, if ever, the baby had previously been fed. (Pathology; 1 to 2 days; Application; Difficulty 4)

117. The answer is C. Menstrual irregularities and pain are not known to be related to whether the woman breastfed her children. (Immunology; Preconception; Knowledge; Difficulty 2)

118. The answer is D. Direct breastfeeding is the norm. All other feeding methods are considered interventions with known and unknown consequences. (Legal; General Principles; Knowledge; Difficulty 3)

119. The answer is D. Even though amoxicillin is considered compatible with breastfeeding, the infant may develop diarrhea or loose stools. (Pharmacology; 4 to 6 months; Knowledge; Difficulty 4)

120. The answer is D. Alcohol in milk is directly related to levels in maternal serum and does not accumulate in milk. (Pharmacology; General Principles; Knowledge; Difficulty 4)

121. The answer is A. Taking birth control pills is not likely to have caused sudden-onset sore nipples. The other questions are appropriate. This mother had a bacterial infection, probably related to the fact that several family members had strep throat. (Pharmacology; 7 to 12 months; Application; Difficulty 2)

122. The answer is C. There is no evidence of increased dental caries from nighttime breastfeeding in the second year of life. The child who nurses past 12 months of age receives substantial immune protection, nutrition, and psychological benefits from breastfeeding (Pathology; >12 months; Application; Difficulty 3)

123. The answer is B. This is a plugged nipple pore, also known as a "bleb" or "white spot." (Pathology; 1 to 3 months; Application; Difficulty 3)

124. The answer is B. This nipple wound was caused by a baby with tongue-tie (short and/or tight lingual frenulum). Normal breastfeeding does not cause this kind of wound; shallow latch is unlikely to cause this much damage in just 8 days, and an 8-day-old is unlikely to be biting during feeds. (Pathology; 3 to 14 days; Knowledge; Difficulty 3)

125. The answer is B. The bulge is a galactocele. Plugged ducts are rarely visible on the breast surface. Inflammation is characteristic of both mastitis and abscess. (Pathology; 3 to 14 days; Knowledge; Difficulty 5)

126. The answer is C. The baby has a short, tight frenulum, which might interfere with effective breastfeeding. However, direct breastfeeding is the ultimate goal and the normative behavior to reinforce. Not all babies with tight frenula will have a problem breastfeeding. If direct breastfeeding is ineffective or painful, options A, B, or D could be considered. (Pathology; 1 to 2 days; Application; Difficulty 4)

127. The answer is D. This baby is tongue-tied. Frenotomy (incision of the lingual frenulum) is a appropriate and effective treatment, especially when ordinary lactation techniques have not been helpful. (Pathology; 3 to 14 days; Application; Difficulty 5)

128. The answer is A. Breast abscesses are usually the result of delayed or inadequate treatment for mastitis. Rarely, physical trauma may precipitate abscess formation. The baby's oral bacteria are not implicated in abscess formation in the lactating breast. (Pathology; 1 to 3 months; Application; Difficulty 4)

129. The answer is D. The child had strep throat, which caused a strep infection of the nipple and the damage shown in this picture. Ordinary breastfeeding does not cause nipple damage. Washing the breasts after every feed is impractical and unnecessary. Biting rarely shows up as the lesion on the areola and crack at the nipple base. (Pathology; 4 to 6 months; Application; Difficulty 4)

130. The answer is A. Paget's disease is a type of nipple cancer and the least likely cause of the small wound shown. The lesion is an unhealed sore caused by the baby's poor suck due to a short frenulum which persisted for $2\frac{1}{2}$ months. (Pathology; 1 to 3 months; Knowledge; Difficulty 5)

131. The answer is D. A mother with a history of sexual abuse should FIRST be encouraged to breastfeed. Only if direct breastfeeding is rejected should pumping be suggested. The other reasons for pumping are appropriate. (Pathology; 3 to 14 days; Application; Difficulty 2)

132. The answer is D. A cleft palate is unlikely to cause the horizontal crack in this mother's nipples. This mother's baby was thrusting his tongue forward to control the mother's oversupply of milk and strong milk ejection reflex. The picture was taken at $2\frac{1}{2}$ weeks postbirth. (Pathology; 15 to 28 days; Application; Difficulty 3)

133. The answer is C. Torticollis is the most likely reason that this baby prefers to turn his head right. Torticollis is an abnormal condition of the neck muscles, especially the sternocleidomastoid. (Pathology; 7, 15 to 28 days; Knowledge; Difficulty 3)

134. The answer is B. This baby has oral thrush, which easily transfers to mother's nipples. Although a mother may have a vaginal candida infection, it is most likely that she will have symptoms of thrush on her nipples. (Pathology; 15 to 28 days; Application; Difficulty 3)

135. The answer is C. There is no research supporting the use of HOT compresses to relieve milk stasis or edema. This woman's chief complaint is the accessory breast tissue in her armpit; her breasts are neither overfull nor swollen, and the baby is nursing well. (Pathology; 3 to 14 days; Application; Difficulty 2)

136. The answer is D. The American Academy of Pediatrics does not recommend routine supplementation of vitamin D in the breastfed infant. Supplementation should be based on history and a case-by-case basis. (Pathology; 4 to 6 months; Application; Difficulty 2)

137. The answer is C. Hypersensitivity reactions to ingested substances rarely include sleepiness. Skin rashes, wheezing, colic, and irritability are all common hypersensitivity reactions. (Pathology; 4 to 6 months; Application; Difficulty 3)

138. The answer is C. Persistent spitting up in the otherwise normal exclusively breastfed baby is most likely an allergic or hypersensitivity response to a substance in mother's diet. Cow's milk is a highly likely cause. And cow's milk allergy may be responsible for up to 42% of gastroesophageal reflux in babies. (Pathology; 4 to 6 months; Knowledge; Difficulty 4)

139. The answer is A. Frequency of sexual intercourse is unrelated to the LAM method (Physiology; 4 to 6 months; Knowledge; Difficulty 2)

140. The answer is B. A common sign of disorganized sucking is that the baby feeds for extended periods with its eyes closed. Thirty to 45 minutes per breast is not normal behavior for this healthy 3-week-old. Mother's milk supply cannot be ascertained by infant feeding behavior, and labor drugs would have mostly cleared by now. (Physiology; 15 to 28 days; Application; Difficulty 5)

141. The answer is D. These lactating breasts are entirely normal. The mother's baby is 13 months old and thriving. A is false. B and C may be true, but cannot be determined solely from breast appearance. (Physiology; >12 months; Application; Difficulty 4)

142. The answer is D. This baby is 4 days old. The milk in the cup is slightly yellow, suggesting transitional milk. The baby's skin is slightly yellow, suggesting mild jaundice, which would be considered pathological if the baby were younger than 3 to 4 days. (Physiology; 3 to 14 days; Application; Difficulty 4)

143. The answer is C. Vigorous pulling and stretching has not been shown to improve breastfeeding success for mothers with flat nipples, and can actually damage tissue. The other actions will support her breastfeeding. (Physiology; Prenatal; Application; Difficulty 2)

144. The answer is B. Feeding the baby and noticing any changes related to milk flow is the FIRST action to take. If the swelling decreases after nursing, it is likely that the accessory breast tissue in the axilla has an outlet. (Physiology; 3 to 14 days; Application; Difficulty 4)

145. The answer is B. Fat content in milk rises as the breast empties, so the proportion of fat from one breast is highest when the baby has fed several times from that breast. (Physiology; 15 to 28 days; Knowledge; Difficulty 4)

146. The answer is D. The Lctation Amenorrhea Method offers the highest (at least 98%) protection against unplanned pregnancy and is the most compatible method with continued breastfeeding. (Physiology; 15 to 28 days; Application; Difficulty 5)

147. The answer is B. Massaging the breast toward the nipple during pumping or feeding helps move milk from the alveoli toward the nipple. (Physiology; 3 to 14 days; Knowledge; Difficulty 4)

148. The answer is B. Facial rashes are a common reaction to cow milk proteins. Direct exposure from artificial baby milk is the most likely trigger. (Immunology; 1 to 3 months; Application; Difficulty 4)

149. The answer is D. The baby's lingual frenulum is short and tight, attached at the tongue tip and on the bottom (alveolar) gum ridge. This prevents the tongue from creating a good seat at breast. (Anatomy; 3 to 14 days; Application; Difficulty 4)

150. The answer is C. This tongue shape is unusual. This baby's other oral anatomic structures are normal. (Anatomy; 1 to 3 months; Application; Difficulty 3)

151. The answer is A. This nipple is somewhat short and flat. After the baby's frenulum was released, he had more success with latch and feeding. The breast is not engorged, and the nipple is in the normal range of sizes. (Anatomy; 3 to 14 days; Application; Difficulty 3)

152. The answer is C. The hypoglossal is the primary motor nerve of the tongue. The other nerves listed are involved in suck-swallow-breathe but play a lesser role in tongue movement. (Anatomy; General Principles; Application; Difficulty 5)

153. The answer is D. This is a normal breast. The slight pink color of the nipple and areola is normal for this woman. (Anatomy; 15 to 28 days; Application; Difficulty 5)

154. The answer is B. The pale-colored lumps on the areola are Montgomery's tubercles (Montgomery's glands) and are completely normal. (Anatomy; >12 months; Application; Difficulty 2)

155. The answer is B. This nipple retracts upon compression at the areola. (Anatomy; Prenatal; Knowledge; Difficulty 5)

156. The answer is B. Small nipples work just fine for breastfeeding. This woman's breast is entirely normal. (Anatomy; Preconception; Application; Difficulty 5)

157. The answer is B. This rash on the baby's thigh is one manifestation of allergic disease. (Immunology; 1 to 3 months; Application; Difficulty 5)

158. The answer is C. The reddened skin is only found on the genitalia and anal opening, suggesting an allergic response. Yeast infections are characterized by blisters or papules. Acidic urine does not result from human milk feedings, and chemical sensitivities would likely appear under the entire diaper area. This baby was in fact allergic to dairy products ingested by her mother. (Immunology; 15 to 28 days; Application; Difficulty 3)

159. The answer is D. This is a bacterial infection of the nipple skin, diagnosed by the mother's doctor. Immediate weaning is not appropriate, because the baby has already been exposed and may even have caused the infection. A nipple shield may provide some comfort, providing it is thoroughly cleaned between uses. Choices A and C are also appropriate. (Immunology; 15 to 28 days; Application; Difficulty 3)

160. The answer is B. On days 1 to 3, the baby gets about 30 ml/day (1 oz/day) of colostrum. As lactogenesis II progresses, the baby obtains more per day as milk volume rapidly rises to about 600 ml/day (20 oz/day) or more by day 5. (Biochemistry; 15 to 28 days; Knowledge; Difficulty 5)

161. The answer is C. The nutritional quality of human milk does NOT diminish at 6 months. The other reasons are legitimate milestones in feeding this healthy 6-month old girl. (Biochemistry; 4 to 6 months; Knowledge; Difficulty 2)

162. The answer is B. Breast shells with wide backs will protect the injured skin from the rubbing of her bra or clothing. (Equipment; 3 to 14 days; Application; Difficulty 3)

163. The answer is C. Tube feeding devices do not correct a dysfunctional sucking pattern. The other answers are appropriate uses. The device pictured is a Medela Supplemental Nursing System. (Equipment; 1 to 3 months; Application; Difficulty 2)

164. The answer is B. A silicone nipple shield is the least helpful of the above suggestions. The sore spot on her nipple tip is very tiny, and most often better positioning and latch will remedy the problem (Equipment; 3 to 14 days; Application; Difficulty 2)

165. The answer is D. Thorough cleaning after each use and sterilization once a day is the most common recommendation by pump manufacturers. (Equipment; 3 to 14 days; Knowledge; Difficulty 5)

166. The answer is C. Breast binders have not been found to be safe or effective for inflammatory conditions of the lactating breast. (Techniques; 3 to 14 days; Application; Difficulty 5)

167. The answer is B. Uneven breast size is very common. Total milk production is not to be related to breast size. (Physiology; 3 to 14 days; Application; Difficulty 4)

168. The answer is C. Nipple thrush often has few visible signs—identification is based on clinical symptoms of itching, stinging, and/or burning. The slightly pink color of her nipples, combined with the sensations reported, is highly suggestive of nipple thrush (candida). (Pathology; 15 to 28 days; Application; Difficulty 5)

169. The answer is C. Moist wound healing is most effective. Choice D is the second-best response. A and D are unhelpful strategies because they dry the skin surface and retard healing. (Techniques; 1 to 2 days; Application; Difficulty 4)

170. The answer is B. The practitioner is performing a frenotomy, an incision of the baby's lingual frenulum, which was short and tight. Frenectomy is removal of tissue, not a simple incision. Tonsillectomy (removal of the tonsils) would have no relationship to the breastfeeding problem, and myringotomy is ear surgery. (Techniques; 3 to 14 days; Application; Difficulty 3)

171. The answer is D. The amount of areola in the mouth is the least important indicator of a problem latch. In this picture, the pursed lips, puckering at the nasolabial crease, and chin failing to touch the breast are all strong indications of a poor latch and positioning. The baby in this picture was tongue-tied. (Techniques; 3 to 14 days; Application; Difficulty 4)

172. The answer is B. Assuring good alignment and deep latch is the FIRST action to take. After that, C would be the next step to take. Nipple tenderness is not normal during any stage of lactation, and referral for evaluation of the tongue musculature would be rarely needed. (Techniques; 15 to 28 days; Application; Difficulty 4)

173. The answer is B. Putting the baby to breast will help the uterus expell the placenta and reduce bleeding. Skilled home birth attendants carry medications to aid uterine contractions for emergency situations. (Physiology; Labor/birth (perinatal); Application; Difficulty 5)

174. The answer is D. The crack at the base of the nipple plus the shiny, reddish skin are common signs of nipple thrush. The other suggestions may provide some relief until the nipple thrush is dealt with. (Techniques; 4 to 6 months; Application; Difficulty 5)

175. The answer is C. Taking a thorough history of the dyad's food intake is the first step in identifying any possible allergic reactions to ingested food or allergens transferred via milk. (Techniques; 4 to 6 months; Application; Difficulty 4)

176. The answer is C. Skin-to-skin contact is the FIRST and least interventive of the strategies suggested, and often the most effective. (Techniques; 1 to 2 days; Application; Difficulty 4)

177. The answer is D. Frequent nursing on the affected side is the FIRST, least complicated approach to opening a plugged nipple pore. C is not appropriate, since the plug is a mechanical problem. B is the next best strategy, with A being the riskiest recommendation. (Techniques; >12 months; Application; Difficulty 4)

178. The answer is C. This is the most accurate description of this baby's tongue. Unseen in the photo is the baby's very short, tight lingual frenulum. (Techniques; 3 to 14 days; Application; Difficulty 4)

179. The answer is A. This 5-month-old exclusively breastfed baby is entirely normal. The teething behavior suggests that she will soon be interested in family foods. (Techniques; 4 to 6 months; Application; Difficulty 3)

180. The answer is B. Early breastfeeding is the most important action when a mother has flat nipples or, for that matter, for all mothers. Prenatal nipple preparation has not been shown to significantly improve flat nipples. (Techniques; Prenatal; Application; Difficulty 3)

181. The answer is C. The mother is doing a digital oral assessment to feel her baby's palate. This also explains why she is not wearing gloves. (Techniques; 3 to 14 days; Knowledge; Difficulty 4)

182. The answer is B. Observing a full breastfeeding is always recommended and appropriate, especially before more complicated assessment is done. (Techniques; 7 to 12 months; Application; Difficulty 5)

183. The answer is A. Correcting positioning and latch is the most important strategy to increase nipple comfort during breastfeeding. In this mother's case, deeper attachment significantly reduced pain; treating the mild thrush infection removed the remaining discomfort. (Techniques; 1 to 2 days; Application; Difficulty 5)

184. The answer is A. The NCHS growth charts were developed based on babies received mixed feeds, not exclusively breastfed infants. New charts based on the healthy, breastfed baby are in development. This 4-month old boy is normal in every way. (Research; 4 to 6 months; Application; Difficulty 5)

185. The answer is B. The pump flange was too small in diameter for this mother's large, fibrous nipples. (Pathology; 1 to 2 days; Application; Difficulty 4)

186. The answer is B. Breastfed twins often are best friends and copy each other's breastfeeding behaviors. High milk volume may increase mother's susceptibility to milk stasis. (Psychology; 7 to 12 months; Application; Difficulty 2)

187. The answer is C. An empathetic response that clarifies the mother's feelings is the first step to establishing rapport in a counseling situation. After the mother's feelings are clearly identified, then solutions can be addressed. (Psychology; 7 to 12 months; Application; Difficulty 3)

188. The answer is D. Mothers talking one-to-one to other mothers has been shown to be an effective strategy for supporting breastfeeding since at least the 1920s. (Psychology; General Principles; Knowledge; Difficulty 5)

189. The answer is A. Breastfeeding cannot be forced on a child at any age. The child who does not want to breastfeed will either bite or refuse to latch on. The other reasons are all common reasons for continued breastfeeding well into the second year of the child's life. (Psychology; >12 months; Application; Difficulty 2)

190. The answer is A. Most babies continue waking at night for feeding throughout the first year of life, and may get up to one third of their calories at night. (Psychology; 4 to 6 months; Application; Difficulty 4)

191.   The answer is B. This child is 6 months old and has been experimenting with self-feeding. (Growth; 4 to 6 months; Application; Difficulty 4)

192.   The answer is D. Most cultures protect and support the new mother for several weeks postbirth, which facilitates the mother's reentry into the community. (Psychology; Labor/birth (perinatal): Application; Difficulty 2)

193.   The answer is D. Stools are usually more formed because of milk composition and addition of family foods. (Growth; 7 to 12 months; Application; Difficulty 4)

194.   The answer is B. One- to 3-month-old exclusively breastfed babies usually do not have long stretches without breastfeeding, even at night. (Growth; 1 to 3 months; Application; Difficulty 2)

195.   The answer is A. Many babies show signs of developmental readiness around 6 months of age, such as reaching for family foods. Exclusive breastfeeding is recommended for at least 6 months. (Growth; 4 to 6 months; Application; Difficulty 4)

196.   The answer is D. The over-1-year old nursing child often plays and explores mother's body during breastfeeding sessions. (Growth; >12 months; Application; Difficulty 5)

197.   The answer is C. Distractibility is common in the 4 to 6 month period. The baby is usually not yet developmentally ready for solid foods at this time. (Growth; 4 to 6 months; Application; Difficulty 2)

198.   The answer is B. In the quiet alert state, the baby's eyes are open, arms extended and relaxed, hands loosely open. The baby's expression is calm and relaxed. (Growth; 15 to 28 days; Knowledge; Difficulty 4)

199.   The answer is C. This 13-month-old's nursing pattern is entirely normal. (Growth; >12 months; Knowledge; Difficulty 3)

200.   The answer is A. Competition with the baby's own mother is highly unlikely. This picture shows the author carrying her perfectly normal, wonderful, gorgeous, and brilliant granddaughter at about 4 weeks of age. (Psychology; 15 to 28 days; Knowledge; Difficulty 2)